Hippocratic Oratory

On Ancient Medicine, *On the Art*, *On Breaths*, *On the Nature of Human Beings* and *On the Sacred Disease* are among the most well-known and sophisticated works of the Hippocratic Collection. The authors of these treatises were seeking means to express their arguments that built on authoritative models of their predecessors. By examining the range of expressive resources used in their expository prose, James R. Cross demonstrates how oral tradition and written techniques, such as sound patterning, signposting and antithetical formulae, were deployed to help the writers develop a case. The book demonstrates that there were various layers of meaning and manners of communicating ideas which can be found in Hippocratic expository prose, and offers fresh insights into the oral debating culture and experiments in persuasion which characterise the ancient Greek world of the late fifth century BCE.

James R. Cross is a Tutor in Classical Civilisation at University College London. He completed his PhD in Classics at King's College London. His research focuses on connections between ancient medicine and literature.

Medicine and the Body in Antiquity
Series Editor: Patricia Baker, University of Kent, UK

Series Advisory Board
Lesley A. Dean-Jones, University of Texas at Austin, USA
Rebecca Gowland, University of Durham, UK
Jessica Hughes, Open University, UK
Ralph Rosen, University of Pennsylvania, USA
Kelli Rudolph, University of Kent, UK

Medicine and the Body in Antiquity is a new series which aims to foster inter-disciplinary research that broadens our understanding of past beliefs about the body and its care. The intention of the series is to use evidence drawn from diverse sources (textual, archaeological, epigraphic) in an interpretative manner to gain insights into the medical practices and beliefs of the ancient Mediterranean. The series approaches medical history from a broad thematic perspective that allows for collaboration between specialists from a wide range of disciplines outside ancient history and archaeology such as art history, religious studies, medicine, the natural sciences and music. The series will also aim to bring research on ancient medicine to the attention of scholars concerned with later periods. Ultimately this series provides a forum for scholars from a wide range of disciplines to explore ideas about the body and medicine beyond the confines of current scholarship.

Hippocratic Oratory

The Poetics of Early Greek Medical Prose

James R. Cross

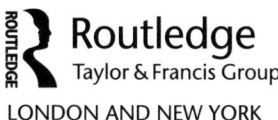

Routledge
Taylor & Francis Group

LONDON AND NEW YORK

First published 2018 by Routledge

2 Park Square, Milton Park, Abingdon, Oxfordshire OX14 4RN

52 Vanderbilt Avenue, New York, NY 10017

Routledge is an imprint of the Taylor & Francis Group, an informa business

First issued in paperback 2020

British Library Cataloguing-in-Publication Data
A catalogue record for this book is available from the British Library

Library of Congress Cataloging-in-Publication Data
Names: Cross, James (James Roger), 1981- author.
Title: Hippocratic oratory : the poetics of early Greek medical prose /
James Cross.
Description: Milton Park, Abingdon, Oxon ; New York, NY :
Routledge, 2018. | Series: Medicine and the body in antiquity | Includes
bibliographical references and index.
Identifiers: LCCN 2017027527| ISBN 9781472474155 (hardback :
alkaline paper) | ISBN 9781315611181 (ebook)
Subjects: LCSH: Medicine, Greek and Roman--History--Sources. |
Medical literature--Greece--Criticism, Textual. | Hippocrates--Influence. |
Hippocrates. Works. | Greek prose literature, Hellenistic--Criticism,
Textual. | Oratory, Ancient--History and criticism. | Oral tradition--
Greece--History--To 1500. | Debates and debating--Greece--History--
To 1500. | Poetics--History--To 1500.
Classification: LCC R138 .C76 2018 | DDC 610.938--dc23
LC record available at https://lccn.loc.gov/2017027527

ISBN: 978-1-4724-7415-5 (hbk)
ISBN: 978-0-367-59410-7 (pbk)

Typeset in Times New Roman
by Sunrise Setting Ltd, Brixham, UK

Contents

Acknowledgements

It is my pleasure to acknowledge those who have contributed to the writing of this book, which began as a PhD thesis at King's College London.

I would firstly like to thank my literature, history and Latin teachers at the Midlands school and sixth form college which I attended. They first inspired in me a serious interest in the written word and the roots of things. I realise how very fortunate I was to have been offered the opportunity to study Latin at a state school.

It was a great privilege to be accepted to study English Literature as an undergraduate at University College London; the invaluable lessons I learnt about literature in this department have guided me ever since.

I would like to thank Emma Dench, who was an important source of inspiration while I was working towards an MA in Classical Civilisation at Birkbeck College, University of London, both for encouraging me to continue studying Classics and for pointing me in the direction of Antonio de Freitas – who has been a friend and source of fascinating conversations ever since – and Rebecca Flemming, with whom I first discussed the PhD project on ancient Greek medical writing and who became my second thesis supervisor.

I am very grateful to Michael Trapp at King's College London, who was my first and main thesis supervisor, for taking on the project and seeing through its development to successful completion as well as for continued insightful comments on my work. As a PhD student at King's, I received financial support from the Leverhulme Trades Charities Trust and from the University College London Study Assistance Scheme.

Rosalind Thomas' and Serafina Cuomo's comments during my thesis *viva* helped me to tighten up my arguments and challenged me to express my ideas more clearly and support them more thoroughly. More recently, Elizabeth Craik has read and offered useful comments on draft versions of this book.

I am grateful to the anonymous reviewers of the proposal and drafts of this book and to Patricia Baker, the Series Editor and Michael Greenwood, Editor at Routledge, for their assistance in bringing the book to publication. Christine Walsh, Maya Davies and my father helped with proofreading at various stages.

I am also grateful to the staff of the Institute of Classical Studies and the Wellcome Library in London for assistance at various points and for providing wonderful places in which to think and meet many like-minded people, including Anastasia Lazani who helped me with learning Greek.

Many thanks also to Christine Hoffmann and my colleagues as well as the students I have taught at the University College London Centre for Language and International Education for providing a congenial and intellectually engaging atmosphere in which to write this book.

Finally, I would like to thank most of all my parents, Jean and Roger – both health professionals – and my brother, Matthew.

Abbreviations and editions

I refer to the Greek text of the five Hippocratic treatises focused on in this study as printed in the following editions. Note that other editions of these treatises show different line and section numbering and minor differences in the Greek.

Jouanna, J. (ed. and trans.) (2003), *Hippocrate. Tome II, 3e partie. La maladie sacrée* Paris: Les Belles Lettres.

Jouanna, J. (ed. and trans.) (2002 [1975]), *Corpus Medicorum Graecorum I, 1, 3. Hippocrate. La nature de l'homme*. Berlin: Akademie-Verlag.

Jouanna, J. (ed. and trans.) (1988), *Hippocrate. Tome V, 1re partie. Des vents; De l'art*. Paris: Les Belles Lettres.

Mann, J. E. (2012), *Hippocrates, On the Art of Medicine*. Leiden; Boston: Brill.

Schiefsky, M. (2005), *Hippocrates: On Ancient Medicine*. Leiden; Boston: Brill.

I rely on the English and French translations of the Greek in the editions listed above and below to produce English translations of extracts from the Hippocratic treatises referred to in this book.

Jones, W. H. S. (ed. and trans.) (1923-1931 [reprinted 1998-2005]), *Hippocrates I-IV*. Cambridge, Mass.; London, England: Harvard University Press.

Jouanna, J. (ed. and trans.) (1990), *Hippocrate. Tome II, 1re partie. De l'ancienne médicine*. Paris: Les Belles Lettres.

I make use of the following abbreviations in referring to texts of the Pre-Socratics and Sophists, where applicable, and cite the Greek text as printed in TEGP, except where indicated. I have generally also cited D. W. Graham's English translations of Pre-Socratic and Sophistic texts, except where indicated.

DK Diels, H. and Kranz, W. (ed. and trans.) (1964), *Die Fragmente der Vorsokratiker: griechisch und deutsch*. Zurich; Berlin, Weidmann.

TEGP Graham, D. W. (2010), *The Texts of Early Greek Philosophy: the Complete Fragments and Selected Testimonies of the Major Pre-Socratics*. Cambridge: Cambridge University Press.

1   Hippocratic expository prose

Introduction

This study is concerned with the poetics and persuasive function of a group of treatises in the Hippocratic Collection which shows signs of being composed for or in relation to oral dissemination and which, as such, should be considered as evidence for Hippocratic oratory.[1] The focus in this study is principally on five of these 'oral' Hippocratic treatises: *On Ancient Medicine* (*De vetere medicina*), *On the Art* (*De arte*), *On Breaths* (*De flatibus*), *On the Sacred Disease* (*De morbo sacro*) and *On the Nature of Human Beings* (*De natura hominum*), which are all believed to have been written towards the end of the fifth century in Greece during a period of seismic cultural, intellectual and social change in the ancient Greek world. These treatises were deeply implicated in these changes and should be valued for the insights they can offer into fifth-century debating culture and their affinity with the developing body of prose writing broadly understood, as much as for their medical content and relationship with other Hippocratic treatises.

My argument is essentially that these Hippocratic works represent significant examples not only of developments in medical understanding and philosophical debate about the nature of the human body and its ailments, but also valuable evidence for the early development of prose writing in ancient Greece: reading the 'oral' Hippocratic treatises as evidence for experiments in authoritative persuasion and creative exercises in explanation in the relatively new form of expository prose yields fresh insights into the volatile and exciting world of late fifth-century oratory that have yet to be explored fully in existing scholarship. My main interest lies in how, in the selected Hippocratic treatises, language is used to make sense of the world, and how language use to an extent *interacts* with – that is, shapes and reflects – these authors' understanding of the workings of the human body, of disease development and so on.

I focus on the persuasive function of recurring patterns in language use: for example, antitheses and balancing effects in phrasing, repetitions and accumulations of words or phrases, tags and sonic effects such as rhyme or resonance in sound, as well as key items of vocabulary. Many of these are features more commonly associated with poetry than prose; one aim of this book is to elicit and analyse the main poetic features of Hippocratic treatises intended for oral dissemination and consider their persuasive role in pseudo-scientific prose tracts as part of the gradual development from oral poetic models of authoritative account to written prosaic models, which is a strong trend throughout the fifth century BCE and has its roots in developments in previous centuries.

Another, related aim is analysis of the extent to which suggested, accumulated, resonant meanings that emerge through various patterns in the prose overlap with or are entangled with the fast-developing hard logic of philosophical authority that could be said to culminate in Aristotle's *Organon*, written in the fourth century BCE, which can be viewed as an extreme example of the expression of authority through the form of prose. In other words, this study explores the presence of different layers of meaning and modes of 'reasoning' in certain Hippocratic treatises, that are beyond the 'logical' surface content of any given treatise.

I have selected these five treatises from the Hippocratic Collection to focus on because they are among the most similar in style and tone to other philosophical and sophistic writing of the period. As Iain Lonie notes, writing on literacy and the Hippocratic Collection, regarding these essayistic treatises, 'They are rationalisitic, bold in hypothesis, ingenious in argument, sceptical of received opinion, and they share the general commitment to intellectual analysis' (Lonie 1983: 149). Others could easily be included in this study; however, this selection ensures a manageable focus for the close reading of persuasive techniques and allows for discussion of the more prominent persuasive features, as well as hopefully providing an opening for further research on this topic in the future.

I give a brief synopsis of these five treatises in the Appendix to this volume. I turn now to an overview of the Hippocratic Collection and scholars' reaction to expository prose in the Collection, and then introduce the many important influences that lie in the background to composition of such texts and their place within the story of the development of early Greek prose writing.

Medical oratory in the Hippocratic Collection

The Hippocratic Collection contains around seventy treatises. The majority are believed to have been composed in the late fifth and early fourth centuries BCE, though some are likely to have been written as early as 450 BCE and others as late as 250 BCE in different locations around the Mediterranean world.[2]

The Collection in the form in which it exists today can be traced back to the publication of an edition printed in Italy in 1526. Vivian Nutton notes that

> the Aldine press in Venice printed the first edition of the complete works of Hippocrates in Greek, for no single ancient manuscript surviving

today contains every tract from the collection, and many have only a small selection. But it is also clear from the manuscripts themselves and from the work of ancient commentators and compilers of Hippocratic dictionaries that the great majority of the texts printed in 1526 were already circulating together under the name of Hippocrates by the first century AD, if not 300 years earlier.

(2013 [2004]: 60)

The most recent modern editor and translator of the entire Collection, Maximilien Paul Emile Littré (1801–1881) believed the compilation of the treatises into a single Collection took place in Alexandria, noting that 'The Hippocratic Collection did not exist in an authentic manner until after the time of Herophilus [of Alexandria, 335–380 BCE] and his pupils' and believed that most of the treatises of the Collection came to Alexandria from family or medical libraries (Littré 1973 [1839]: vol. 1, 262–291).[3] Nutton also notes that

it [is] likely that the collection was first assembled in broadly the form we have it at Alexandria in Egypt in the famous library of the Ptolemies, at a time when Cos was part of their empire . . . The somewhat haphazard way in which materials were brought together and stored at the Alexandrian library would . . . explain, at least in part, the varied nature of the collection.

(2013 [2004]: 61)

There is only limited and often fanciful evidence available to take us any further than Littré's sense of a body of work formed somewhat haphazardly in the library at Alexandria. Between them, Jody Pinault's edition and translation of fascinating hagiographic-style stories that gathered around the name Hippocrates in *Hippocratic Lives and Legends* and Wesley Smith's edition and translation of letters associated with Hippocrates collect all the relevant sources and attest to the murkiness of our historical knowledge regarding the original composition and dissemination of the treatises of the Collection, as well as the rich body of legends that built up around the name of Hippocrates.[4] If there is no way to be sure precisely when and where the Collection was formed, the internal evidence nevertheless suggests that there were sub-collections of treatises such as the case studies of *Epidemics* or the series of medical maxims entitled *Aphorisms* which are likely to have been grouped prior to being included in the full Collection (see Nutton 2013 [2004]: 61–62). Furthermore, from analysis of the style and content of individual treatises, in relation to what is known about their intellectual or cultural context, scholars can establish probable dates of composition, though in certain cases only an imprecise range of decades or even centuries can be provided; occasional references to other datable historical events or characters – such as the Pre-Socratic philosopher Melissos, in the case of *On the Nature of Human Beings* – also help with dating (Jouanna 2002 [1975]: 59–61).

All the treatises are connected, by manuscripts, with the historical figure Hippocrates. Beyond the name, only the slightest secure information about the identity of Hippocrates exists, though long-standing threads of discussions now referred to as the 'The Hippocratic Question' have been pursued regarding which, if any, of the treatises in the Collection were composed by Hippocrates, and indeed who he was.[5] The Collection was clearly composed by many different hands.

The treatises of the Collection are medical in the loose sense that they all discuss the functions and malfunctions of the human body, yet the Collection also contains much that could be considered ethnographic, historical and above all philosophical rather than solely medical. To take some representative examples, there are treatises that focus on the fundamental causes of diseases; there are those that discuss in detail the therapy that must be applied to cure individual diseases; others explore dietetics, that is the treatment and prevention of diseases by the regulation of daily routines such as eating and drinking habits and frequency, type and level of physical exercise; some treatises contain case histories of patients; others discuss the principles of surgery; another area considered is pregnancy and diseases of women; the Hippocratic oath is one treatise in the Collection that famously discusses medical ethics.

There is an impressive and fascinating treasury of material here that has from antiquity up to the present day been of interest to those studying medicine and to historians of medicine.

In the last forty years or so the Hippocratic Collection has also begun to receive serious critical attention from Classicists from a variety of intellectual backgrounds and so the context of the collection has been explored in greater detail and from a diverse set of perspectives.

Many of the medical writers discuss ideas that reveal an intimate connection with Pre-Socratic and Platonic thought, for example. Connections with discussion of natural philosophy in Herodotus' *Histories* have also provided a rich source for recent research.[6] Ideas central to Hippocratic medicine, such as the notion of humouralism, enshrined as canonical through Galen's high regard for the theory as described in *On the Nature of Human Beings*, shows close links with Alcmaeon of Croton's notion of *isonomia*, of balance of powers, as well as with Empedocles' notions of competing forces in the world at large which need to be balanced. Indeed, many Hippocratic treatises display interests and discuss issues which go beyond understanding of the human body to understanding nature and culture. *Airs, Waters, Places* is an important example of this, which contains analysis of climate and its effects on the body as well as theories of climate and racial difference.[7]

Until recently, however, the Collection has been largely overlooked as evidence for the development of prose. The Hippocratic Collection is widely acknowledged to represent a transformation in the understanding of the body and its place in the natural world as gleaned from early extant Greek writing, such as the Homeric poems in which gods rather than bodily constituents such as phlegm or bile are described as bringing about disease.[8] Yet, it is much less commonly acknowledged in Hippocratic scholarship that along with this deep change in understanding, the language being used to communicate new ideas was relatively untried and itself in the process of rapid development; use of prose represented a fundamental departure from Homeric hexameter and the authority of inspired, poetic voice, and went hand-in-hand with the conceptual changes that were taking place in the period.

One reason for this is perhaps that the treatises of the Collection all too often do not fit easily into the notion of 'classical' in the sense of 'first-class' literary compositions in the way that Plato's dialogues or Thucydides' historiography do and so have attracted only limited attention from scholars interested in issues of form and style. Another explanation may be that their medical content has until recently meant that Hippocratic treatises have been treated as specialised and therefore not of mainstream interest, though this situation is changing.

Of most importance for this study are the areas of cross-fertilisation between the Hippocratic Collection and sophistic authors, which are relevant to the study of the development of prose expression. Until recently, many scholars dismissed sophistic traits of the Hippocratic writings as unimportant, even somewhat dangerous, rather in the same way that we find negative reactions to writers considered Sophists among ancient commentators. This is almost certainly the reason why discussion of the interrelation between Hippocratic and Sophistic oratory has been limited until the last few decades.[9]

Jones, working in the first half of the twentieth century, wrote of the Hippocratic treatise *On Breaths*: 'The author shows no genuine interest in medicine, nor do his contentions manifest any serious study of physiology or pathology' (1923: 222), though he adds that 'We may laugh at the crudities of περὶ φυσῶν . . . but we must respect its inquiring spirit and its restless curiosity' (1923: 223). He calls *On Breaths* a 'sophistic essay, probably written to be delivered to an audience' (1923: 221).

Of *On the Art*, a defence of the art of medicine included within the Hippocratic Collection, which is commonly thought to show intense sophistic influence, Jones writes:

> It is quite plain from even a cursory reading of the treatise that its author was not a physician. His interest lies in subtle reasonings and in literary style, not in science. Besides this, in the last chapter he speaks of 'those

who are skilled in the art' as giving a proof of the existence of medicine based on works, and not, like the proofs given in the present book, on words. He evidently distinguishes himself from medical men.

(1923: 187)

He continues:

The two most striking characteristics of *The Art* are an attenuated logic and a fondness for sophistic rhetoric. The rhetorical character of the whole book is so striking that without doubt it must be attributed to a sophist. The elaborate parallels, verbal antitheses, and balancing of phrase with phrase, can have no other explanation.

(1923: 187)

The label 'sophist', is, for Jones, an indication of want of medical expertise.

By contrast, a more recent editor of these texts acknowledges them as written by doctors in the Hippocratic spirit as well as showing strong sophistic influence. Jouanna writes of *On the Art*:

Neither the sophistic form of the speech, nor the associations with the theories of Diogenes of Apollonia or Empedocles should mask a more profound reality: the treatise has its roots in Hippocratic medicine in the broad sense of the term. It is wrong to view this treatise as the speech of a Sophist mislaid in the Hippocratic Collection. By the tone, the general themes regarding the art of medicine and the detail of its physiological explanations, the work is in accordance with common foundations of Hippocratic medicine.

(1988: 30)[10]

For Jouanna, this treatise is Hippocratic and medical in the deepest sense and should not be considered a sophistic speech extraneous to the main Collection; here, too, though, we can detect a sense that the word 'sophistic' carries negative connotations of superficial or specious.

On *On the Art*, Jouanna writes:

The treatise *On the Art* presents analogies in form with *On Breaths*. It is also an epideictic speech composed with sophistic technique by a physician who is arguing a case. However, the argument is very different: while the author of *On Breaths* claims that air is the cause of all diseases, the author of *On the Art* claims that medicine exists in so far as it is a τέχνη – an 'art'.

(1988: 167)[11]

This treatise is considered as an epideictic speech composed with sophistic techniques by a doctor; there is, here too, a certain distancing from the dangers of the label of sophistry.

There are many treatises in the Collection that are intensely engaged with the spirit of the age in which they were written and, as prose writings, emerge in an unstable interface between poetic and prosaic, oral and literate. In places, some treatises go so far as to begin to develop new modes of expression; this is a phenomenon which echoes contemporary exploration of the possibilities of the expression of meaning in language. This book aims to contribute to the movement in current scholarship examining Hippocratic writings in context and consider the value of these treatises as examples of early Greek prose writing and in terms of their poetics and persuasive function. Unlike some previous scholarship, however, the aim here is to examine behind the negative and dismissive reactions and listen in to the voices of the authors of the most outlandish and performative treatises of the Hippocratic Collection; it seeks to ask what effects they intended to achieve on their audiences and how they went about this, reserving judgement about the effectiveness of their techniques.

Models of Hippocratic medical oratory

In classical Athens, in the fifth century BCE, and across the Greek world culturally and intellectually in touch with Athens' influence, experience and skill in the art of communicating to a live audience was a central and vital feature of everyday life which would have involved all (male, Athenian) citizens, if not all people in Athens, at some level. The democratic assemblies which drew crowds of several thousands were sustained by public eloquence. The establishment of dramatic festivals at Athens, attended by large audiences from across the Greek world, and the development of tragic and comic drama celebrated mastery of the voice, and drew self-conscious attention to dialogue and declamation, spoken and sung. The law courts at Athens, from which most of our evidence for ancient Greek law derives, were driven by the speeches of prosecutors, defendants and witnesses.[12] Public oratorical contests and performances were not only a feature of democratic processes, legal systems and the theatre; the influence of the performance culture of the spoken word extended well into the world of early Greek philosophy and the sciences, including medicine.

No area of cultural or intellectual life was untouched by the pressing need to find ways to communicate ideas in a public forum, before a crowd, in one form or another, in this century of cultural and intellectual revolutions. The evidence of essays designed for public dissemination from the Hippocratic Collection shows that many doctors were certainly part of this impulse towards oratory. In order to gain a sense of the nature of Hippocratic oratory, it is useful to consider its possible genealogy; for, as with other forms of oratory indicated above – in the law courts, in democratic assemblies, in the theatre – it emerges from a tradition of public debate, and specifically public debate on medical topics, for which we have some evidence. The work of several Pre-Socratic thinkers offers some of the earliest evidence for medical oratory extant from Greece, and is likely to have served as a model from which Hippocratic oratory develops.

Empedocles, for example, at the peak of his activities in the mid-fifth century BCE wrote in dactylic hexameter, the metre of Homeric and Hesiodic epic; his work was modelled on epic poetry designed for performance, recited by itinerant professional bards. In terms of form, his work looks back to the epic tradition. The content of his work, however, which focuses on questions of natural philosophy – such as the fundamental structure of the cosmos – rather than mythic narratives, shows a radical departure from the Homeric and Hesiodic tradition.

As a natural philosopher engaged in opening new intellectual territory in verse, there is a general sense in which Empedocles is a direct predecessor of Hippocratic public discussion about the nature of medicine, since his philosophical interests included medical topics.[13] The *Suda* and Diogenes Laertius (8.77) indicate that Empedocles wrote on the topics of physiology such as respiration and embryology (see e.g. TEGP 386–387 (127 [F78])); TEGP 388–389 (130 [F80]), (132 [F82]), (134 [F84]) = DK31B65, B67, B68) and more broadly on nature and on purification, and Galen (*Method of Healing* 1.1, 10-5-6 K) includes Empedocles in a list of early physicians.

Indeed, evidence for Empedocles' work shows an intellectual engaged in two strands of thinking, the interconnection and interplay between which will be the focus of this study on Hippocratic oratory in the late fifth century BCE, as follows: (i) experimentation with different ways of communicating ideas; (ii) concurrent engagement with and development of medical theories.

In the following extract, Empedocles describes himself travelling from city to city where he is revered by people seeking to hear his healing words; he specifically entwines themes of language and healing:

> τοῖσιν ἅμ' εὖτ' ἂν ἵκωμαι ἄστεα τηλεθάοντα,
> ἀνδράσιν ἠδὲ γυναιξί, σεβίζομαι· οἱ δ' ἅμ' ἕπονται
> μυρίοι ἐξερέοντες, ὅπηι πρὸς κέρδος ἀταρπός,
> οἱ μὲν μαντοσυνέων κεχρημένοι, οἱ δ' ἐπὶ νούσων
> παντοίων ἐπύθοντο κλυεῖν εὐηκέα βάξιν,
> δηρὸν δὴ χαλεπῆισι πεπαρμένοι <ἀμφ' ὀδύνηισιν>.

> When I come to other flourishing cities
> I am revered by them, men and women alike; they follow together

by thousands inquiring the path to success,
some seeking oracles, some seeking
to hear the healing word for all sorts of diseases,
having been long pierced by severe <pains>.

(TEGP 406–407 ([F120]) = DK31B112)

Empedocles portrays himself as a religious healer with powers to cure many kinds of diseases through his insights. This is a model of an author's self-representation as saviour, using language that is drawn from the epic past to introduce and discuss topics that relate to everyday health problems; as a saviour-figure, Empedocles also implies that he is able to dispense 'healing words'. While the level of self-fashioning and the tendency to draw on religious and epic themes in this extract does not correlate directly with what is found in Hippocratic expository prose, as will be seen in the following chapters of this study, there is a clear sense of a model here for Hippocratic treatises such as *On Breaths* which communicate the heroism of doctors and which include poetic effects in language to convey both medical theories and the healing power of such theories.

Added to this conjunction of healing and the use of persuasive powers, it is important to note that Empedocles was thought to have reflected on the topic of persuasion and be involved with the development theories of eloquence too. Quintilian, the first-century CE Roman author on rhetoric, notes that

> Empedocles is said to be the first one after those poets referred to, to promote anything about rhetoric. The earliest writers of textbooks [on rhetoric], Corax and Tisias were from Sicily, followed by Gorgias of Leontini, a man of the same island, who was, as it is reported, a student of Empedocles.
>
> (TEGP 338–339 (12) = DK31A19)[14]

This development of rhetorical handbooks goes beyond anything we find evidence for in the writers of Hippocratic oratory; nevertheless, they too were involved the development and promotion of new techniques of persuasion, as well as in discussions of medical theory.

Other Pre-Socratic philosophers, such as Xenophanes and Heraclitus, have no demonstrable connection with specifically medical topics but as natural philosophers engaged in the development and use of new modes of expression, they almost certainly played a part in sparking and influencing the emergence of public debates on medical topics. Their work seeks to develop new philosophical ideas partly *alongside* and *through* experimentation with language use; this manner of thinking and expressing at the same time on topics relating to natural philosophy was of significant and demonstrable influence on several key Hippocratic writers. Detailed discussion of links between Heraclitus and *On Breaths* follows in Chapter 4 of this book.

Xenophanes, a forebear of Parmenides and Empedocles, was known in antiquity as a wandering performer and poet, and had interests in cosmogony and astronomy, nature and divinity. The religious tone of Xenophanes' style of communication and references to pious behaviour show one way in which the author both indicates and embodies his interests in the divine as part of his enquiries into the nature of divine, as, for example, in the following: 'χρὴ δὲ πρῶτον μὲν θεὸν ὑμνεῖν εὔφρονας ἄνδρας / εὐφήμοις μύθοις καὶ καθαροῖσι λόγοις' 'It is right for men of good will to hymn the god first of all, / with auspicious tales and pure words' (TEGP 102–103 (9 [F1]) = DK21B1). Here, Xenophanes recommends expressing reverence for the divine in hymns. At the same time, elsewhere in his poem, he is offering his audience a new kind of religious poetry in which he proceeds to express his own version of understanding of the divine, which includes questioning the behaviour of the gods: he notes that the gods are considered by some to be the source of all that is blameworthy and disgraceful among mortals (TEGP 108–109 (29 [F17]) = DK21B11).

In a similar vein, Heraclitus makes use of style of expression in part to engage in philosophical questions about the nature of nature. Throughout antiquity and beyond, Heraclitus' enigmatic style and love of paradox and ambiguity have drawn a range of strong reactions. From Lucretius in the Roman philosophical poem *On the Nature of Things*, composed over four centuries after Heraclitus' death, we have a dismissive reaction to Heraclitus' philosophical contribution:

> quapropter qui materiam rerum esse putarunt
> ignem atque ex igni summam consistere solo,
> magno opere a vera lapsi ratione videntur.
> Heraclitus init quorum dux proelia primus,
> clarus ob obscurum linguam magis inter inanis
> quamde gravis inter Graios qui vera requirunt.
> omnia enim stolidi magis admirantur amantque
> inversis quae sub verbis latitantia cernunt,
> veraque constituunt quae belle tangere possunt
> auris et lepido quae sunt fucata sonore.

Wherefore, those who have thought fire is the matter of things and the totality is composed of fire only have clearly fallen far from the true account. Heraclitus first joined battle as their general, thought brilliant for his dark utterance more among the empty-headed than among serious Greeks who seek the truth. For dimwits admire and love all things which they can discern hidden under twisted words, and they regard as true words that prettily tickle their ears, and are coloured with graceful sound.

(Lucretius *De Rerum Natura*, I. 635–644 = TEGP 182–183 (169))

Heraclitus' 'twisted words' sought to convey complex ideas in natural philosophy. While Lucretius clearly does not take Heraclitus' work seriously, these lines suggest that the Pre-Socratic philosopher did succeed in provoking some manner of public engagement with philosophical ideas; this in turn is a clue to his influence on some of the Hippocratic oratorical texts. Lucretius is, of course, writing over 400 years after Heraclitus' lifetime, but this passage emerges from a tradition of responses to Heraclitus' work which include close contemporaries who found his work befuddling: Aristotle comments, for instance, that Heraclitus' writing does not make logical sense, with all statements being both true and false (TEGP 182–183 (167) = Aristotle *Metaphysics* 1012a24–26, a29–31, a33–b2).[15]

In the work of Xenophanes, Heraclitus, Parmenides and Empedocles, in different ways and to different degrees, we find, then, fragmentary evidence for writing that is likely to have served as models for the kinds of composition designed for public performance found in the Hippocratic Collection. To be clear, the period in which Xenophanes, Heraclitus, Parmenides and Empedocles were working is characterised by two major and interrelated shifts. Firstly, poetry was ceding to prose as the dominant form of authoritative expression on all questions of major intellectual importance. Secondly, a society that relied predominantly on oral expression was evolving into one that placed ever-increasing emphasis on the value of the written word in its records, its forms of self-expression and its enquiries. In order to begin to consider the nature of Hippocratic oratory, these shifts must be acknowledged and considered. I turn now to a brief introduction to and outline of each of them to establish some further background context for the study of Hippocratic oratory.

Poetry and prose in late fifth-century intellectual debates in the Hellenic world

In this section, I offer a brief sketch of some of the main ideas and sources relating to the rise in dominance of written prose and its development. For the purposes of this study, it is important to emphasise the main differences between verse and prose; the point that a contest between authoritative media is underway in fifth century BCE in Greece; and some of the intellectual ramifications of the development of prose as the main form of authoritative communication. I am also interested in pointing out the way in which development of prose style and theories of knowledge and reasoning become entangled in certain ways in this period; this converging relationship between thought and expression is pertinent to the discussion in the following chapters and is a significant feature of Hippocratic oratorical treatises.

Written prose most closely reflects the everyday conversational exchanges that we can presume are a feature of life for all people in all periods of history; it is a form of expression that presents itself as at one with the commonplace comings and goings of everyday life, as the adjective 'prosaic' may imply. Poetry, by contrast, seeks to distinguish itself from the mundane and quotidian, and express something which is not normally expressed, cannot normally be expressed, or is only permitted to be expressed by certain people. The category 'prose' exists only insofar as it is a point of contrast with the category 'poetry' or 'verse'. In the ancient world, as will be explored further in the following chapters, examples of prose on scientific or technical subjects in the ancient Greek world show many 'poetic' elements; in its most fundamental conception, however, poetry must be considered as words written to fit a certain metre which are frequently sung or recited to music. Whatever the degree of 'poetic' elements it embraces, prose in ancient Greek had no regular metre and was not sung or recited to music.[16]

Records exist of statements in list form from the earliest times in the ancient Greek world. The Linear B tablets written in Mycenaean Greek, for instance, contain many lists of records of exchanges of goods. The first records of grammatically connected prose in ancient Greece derive from the late sixth or early fifth century BCE.[17] While written prose was clearly always in use in the ancient world, more intellectually demanding or abstract issues and topics thought more divine were explored and expressed in the Archaic period in ancient Greece in poetic form. To compose an explanation in words of the nature of the universe in the eighth century BCE meant to give an account in poetic form by means of divine inspiration, as we find, for example, with Hesiod's *Theogony*. This is the tradition from which Xenophanes, Parmenides and Empedocles, and to a lesser extent Heraclitus, emerge in the late sixth and early fifth centuries BCE.

Many of the Pre-Socratic philosophers chose not to compose in verse form and here we find one thread of evidence for the movement towards the challenging and dismantling of the authoritative status of poetic metre with its associations of divine inspiration and the development of explanations without metre intended to be accepted as authoritative enquiries into natural philosophy. Indeed, even the poetry of Xenophanes, Parmenides and Empedocles was thought by some to fall short of the standard set by their predecessors and other literary contemporaries:

> non ita tamen Xenophanes aut Parmenides aut Empedocles sive alii quicumque theologi a poesi capti sunt divini viri, sed potius theoriam naturae gaudio amplexi et vitam omnem ad pietatem laudemque deorum

dedicantes optimi quidem viri comperti sunt, poetae tamen non felices: quos oportebat divinitus spiritum sortiri gratiamque de caelo metrum carmen rhythmumque caelestem ac divinum, ut poemata vera relinquerent velut prototypum libri perfectum et pulcrum cunctis exemplar.

Nevertheless neither Xenophanes, Parmenides, Empedocles nor any other theologians, divine men inspired by poetry, [made the gods liars,] but rather joyously embracing the contemplation of nature and dedicating their whole lives to piety and the praise of the gods they revealed themselves to be the best men, though they were not gifted poets. They should have received a divine spirit and metre, melody, and a heavenly, divine rhythm as a gift from heaven so that they might leave true poems as the perfect model of a book and a beautiful example to all.

(TEGP 100–101 (8) = DK21A26)

In this passage from Philo's *On Providence*, handed down to us in Latin translation, the author associates, however implicitly, the decline in poetic skill with lack of divine inspiration. Philo is writing in the Jewish tradition, attempting to combine Jewish and Hellenistic philosophy into a single theological system, and so might be expected to find these Pre-Socratic authors lacking in divine inspiration; nevertheless, the observation tallies with the point that the use of 'less perfect' poetic models, and later prose, emerges most strikingly among the earliest intellectuals who question the divine and enquire into the nature of nature itself, putting faith in their own powers of thought. As Glenn Most argues in his work on the poetics of the Pre-Socratics, the overall context of the decision about how to compose a piece of writing in the fifth century BCE was a contest for authority between verse and prose (Most 1999: 332–362).

Evidence of the emergent use of sophisticated explanatory prose is also famously found in the first historical accounts in Herodotus' *Histories*, Thucydides' *On the Peloponnesian War* and their mythographer predecessors who sought to upset and overturn the mythic histories which had previously dominated in the form of epic poetry. The competition for authority between the new historiographers writing in prose and their poetic predecessors is clear in one of the most famous examples of oratory from the fifth century BCE, recorded – and part-invented – by Thucydides in *On the Peloponnesian War*. First citizen Pericles' exclamation of the power of prose oratory over the epic poetry of the past in his speech commemorating the dead at the end of the first year of the Peloponnesian War is as follows:

μετὰ μεγάλων δὲ σημείων καὶ οὐ δή τοι ἀμάρτυρόν γε τὴν δύναμιν παρασχόμενοι τοῖς τε νῦν καὶ τοῖς ἔπειτα θαυμασθησόμεθα, καὶ οὐδὲν προσδεόμενοι οὔτε Ὁμήρου ἐπαινέτου οὔτε ὅστις ἔπεσι μὲν τὸ αὐτίκα τέρψει, τῶν δ᾽ ἔργων τὴν ὑπόνοιαν ἡ ἀλήθεια βλάψει, ἀλλὰ πᾶσαν μὲν θάλασσαν καὶ γῆν ἐσβατὸν τῇ ἡμετέρᾳ τόλμῃ καταναγκάσαντες γενέσθαι, πανταχοῦ δὲ μνημεῖα κακῶν τε κἀγαθῶν ἀίδια ξυγκατοικίσαντες.

Our power most certainly does not lack for witness: the proof is far and wide, and will make us the wonder of present and future generations. We have no need of a Homer to sing our praises, or of any encomiast whose poetic version may have immediate appeal but then fall foul of the actual truth. The fact is that we have forced every sea and every land to be open to our enterprise, and everywhere we have established permanent memorials of both failure and success.

(2.41)

Thucydides has Pericles state that Athens' greatness is self-evident to all who encounter the city and its inhabitants, with no need of a Homer to sing its praises in verse, that it has hard proof of its achievements which reflect the truth. In one sense, Pericles' speech is also a reflection of this new kind of encomium, a speech to remind its citizens of that greatness which draws upon demonstrable evidence and is composed in the new language of permanent prose. Thucydides' own voice echoes powerfully in the background to this extract: his is a work created as a possession for all time and thus in competition with the longevity and influence of Homeric epic (1.21, 1). We can also find in this speech a Homeric quality, like the hero giving a speech on the battlefield, which is both very old in Athens at the time and very new. The new speech is given by a leading citizen and military general, not a hero, and while it is a speech, it is the *written record* of that speech which is important to Thucydides. There is evidence in this famous moment from classical Athenian history of a heady mixture of both the poetic and the prosaic, as well as a combination of the oral word (the spoken speech) and its written record.

With Thucydides' account of the plague of Athens in 431–430 BCE, and with Herodotus' many references to medical topics – parts of his *Histories* are uncannily similar to the Hippocratic *Airs, Waters, Places*, for example – we find further evidence of the background to the public debates on medical topics, to authors interested in medical questions and in the development of new languages with which to interrogate these questions.[18] For these early historians, too, asking new questions in new ways, and playing a part in medical debates, the content of their enquiries cannot be cleanly extrapolated from the form which they take.

Poetry, with its emphasis on and concern over the aesthetics of expression, tends to value form as equal to or above the prosecution of ideas and to deflect attention away from discussion of ideas (though *narrative* poetry – epic – often does include debate and argument of practical questions, as famously in the first book of Homer's *Iliad*, for instance) as will be described more fully below. Prose generally allows for more emphasis on and control of theoretical content, and makes participation more immediate and less exclusive. Simon Goldhill notes in *The Invention of Prose*: 'The new language of prose – its writing and delivery and interpretation – is absolutely fundamental . . . to the intellectual revolution of the fifth-century enlightenment [and] to the political functioning of the classical city' (Goldhill 2002: 79). This power of prose is due to the fact that, unlike poetry, it encourages and enables inclusive debate and discussion.

Goldhill also notes regarding the law courts:

> To speak in court is to engage in a competitive environment where the jury is fully aware of a speaker's attempts to persuade, and the speakers are aware of the jury's resistance to being convinced, as well as the competition between himself and the other speakers. The courtroom becomes a self-reflexive, self-aware battleground for control over the narrative of *to eikos* – who can claim the most plausible story, who can stake for himself a convincing position, who can best manipulate the insinuation that his opponent is untrustworthy and deceptive.
>
> (Goldhill 2002: 66)[19]

Although this point is made in relation to the law courts in ancient Athens, it has broad application and relates more generally to all uses of prose which seek to set forth a case in the fifth century, in particular to the Pre-Socratics' enquiries just mentioned and including the Hippocratic treatises examined in this book, whose relationship with legal oratory is an area that is ripe for further research. With the arrival of prose as the medium of ideas, suddenly one author is in direct competition with another over the truth of any given issue, and one theory over another.[20]

The development of prose is therefore closely connected with the development of early notions of prosecution of arguments relating to medical theories and scientific method, as it is with the development of all intellectual innovations in this period which question inherited wisdom and see widened participation.

Being a relatively new means of expression, the nature of prose was also still in the process of being established during the fifth century, and its potential as a vehicle for the expression of new ideas was relatively untested. Nowhere is this truer than in the work of Gorgias and the generation of intellectuals who follow him, commonly known as the Sophists and active in Athens. These thinkers are of special importance in this study because of their close relationship with several important examples of Hippocratic oratory, such as *On Breaths* and *On the Art*. Building particularly on the work of their Pre-Socratic contemporaries and predecessors, and influenced too by all the various new forms of literature that were emerging in the fifth-century BCE including historiography, the Sophists were renowned for their intensity of focus on questions of persuasive theory and their experiment with modes of expression.

Cicero in *De Inventione* notes that 'Gorgias of Leontini, who was almost the earliest orator, thought an orator could speak more effectively than anyone about anything' (450b6–c2 (A27)). Though there were of course orators before Gorgias – as any glance through a Homeric epic can show – Cicero's comment reflects the point that the power of language above all else comes to prominence with Gorgias in a way that it had never done before. However, it would be more accurate to say that rather than being the first orator, Gorgias was the first of a new kind of orator in a new world of oratory, a world which is more self-conscious and reflexive on the interplay between form and content than previous generations, and a world which is pushing at the boundaries of previously known modes of communication.

In his mock defence of the mythical Helen of Troy against the charge of initiating the Trojan War, Gorgias includes an encomium to the persuasive power of language which he indicates is one reason to absolve her of the crime: 'εἰ δὲ λόγος ὁ πείσας καὶ τὴν ψυχὴν ἀπατήσας, οὐδὲ πρὸς τοῦτο χαλεπὸν ἀπολογήσασθαι καὶ τὴν αἰτίαν ἀπολύσασθαι ὧδε.' 'But if words persuaded her and deceived her soul, it is not difficult to defend her in this case, and to absolve her from guilt' (TEGP 758–759 (49 [F10]), Section 8 = DK82B11). Gorgias praises language in a way that turns it into an omnipotent deity, and goes on to claim that words have the power to dispel negative emotions and evoke positive ones.[21]

As well as Gorgias, the fragments of the work of Protagoras, Antiphon (one or two people), Prodicus and the collection of anonymous texts including the *Dissoi Logoi*, show a group of intellectuals engaged fervently with experiments in persuasion and questions of the relationship between language and truth. Protagoras is known, for example, to have presented demonstrations of argument and counter-argument – making 'τὸν ἥττω δὲ λόγον κρείττω ποιεῖν' 'the weaker case the stronger' (TEGP 706–707 (27, 28) = DK80A21). With Protagoras, we find evidence for another key aspect of oratory in the Sophistic tradition. Plato remarks of Protagoras in his dialogue of the same name that he is able to make excellent long speeches and to give succinct answers to questions posed to him, and this is a skill possessed by few. (TEGP 696–697 (5) = DK80A7). While it is possible to find examples of philosophical poetry, of elaborately conceived speeches, of the development of new styles of expression to enable greater persuasive powers and even theorising on the nature of persuasion before them, the Sophists bring spontaneity and *ex tempore* response as an addition to the catalogue of persuasive resources available to speakers of all kinds in the late fifth century BCE, a sign of their belief in their powers of persuasion to respond effectively to any situation or issue.

Indeed, Sophistic texts such as Gorgias' *On What-Is-Not* provided a model for how Pre-Socratic issues could be taken up and re-presented in a catchier style and medium for high-profile public display (TEGP 740–746 (38 [F1a]) = DK82B3, TEGP 746–751 (39 [F1b]). Antiphon the Sophist's discussion of the connection between justice and nature serves a similar purpose, as well as linking discussion about nature with more human-centred concerns (TEGP 812–817 (63 [F46a-c]) = DK87B45). Sophistic texts also established public argument as something that could legitimately and interestingly take place outside the limited contexts of deliberative assemblies and law courts: Protagoras' insistence on the relativity of all knowledge, for instance, invites fundamental debate on all issues, not just those related to governance (TEGP 692–703 (1, 16–19 [F1a-e]) = DK80B1).[22]

With the developments in oratory that are sparked by thinkers such as Gorgias and Protagoras, we begin to see eloquence and theories of eloquence becoming more closely entangled. As Leslie Kurke notes in *Aesopic Conversations*, a lucid recent study on the way in which philosophical prose sought to marginalise the influence of popular tradition largely represented by Aesop's *Fables*,

> the fragmentary evidence we have suggests that the Sophists were (among other things) engaged in fairly wild generic and stylistic experimentation at the boundaries between poetry and prose, in a period when the nature and norms of the latter were still very much up for grabs.
>
> (Kurke 2011: 265–266)

The common reaction towards the work of the Sophists in antiquity, however, was dismissive. In *On Lysias*, Dionysius of Halicarnassus, the first century BCE historian and teacher of rhetoric, quotes Plato (*Phaedrus* 238d) in expressing his ambivalence towards Gorgias' experiments in form: 'Clearly Gorgias of Leontini in many cases exhibits an inelegant and bombastic style, sometimes uttering some phrases "not far removed from certain dithyrambs", and of his companions, the circle of Licymnius and Polus do likewise. His poetic and figurative diction influenced the Athenian orators also, as Timaeus says, beginning from the time he came to Athens as an ambassador and dazzled the audience with his public speech' (TEGP 729–730 (5) = DK82A4).[23] Dionysius acknowledges Gorgias' influence here, but judges his style harshly. Interestingly, it is *because* it is rather too similar to poetry that Dionysius considers it defective; this is an indication that by this period, prose had acquired an identity in strong opposition to verse.

Reacting to the spirit of the Sophists, we find Plato, born around 428 BCE, seeking to dominate and take control over philosophical questions of rhetoric and theories of persuasion in several dialogues, including the *Republic, Gorgias* and *Phaedrus*. Yet, though dismissive of the Sophists, throughout his *oeuvre* too we can detect a creative and experimental approach to the most effective mode of expression.

In Plato's *Symposium*, for example, though the work is not directly concerned with questions of eloquence, we find a dialogue of unsettled and experimental exchanges in which a competition of oratorical responses to the question of 'what is the nature of love?' raises further questions about the best *way* to answer such a question and persuade an audience of the philosophical truth, with the characters representing different approaches (tragic playwright, physician, comic playwright, philosopher, lover). Kurke's study (2011), mentioned above, effectively pulls into focus the strangeness of Plato's prose, with its part-poetic effects and blend of myth and dialectic, and its embodiment of the spirit of experiments in persuasion of its time.

It is also no surprise that Plato includes a physician among those invited to give a speech at the gathering depicted in the *Symposium*. Adding to the heady mix of eloquence and theories of eloquence, ideas about medicine were becoming embroiled and explored in new persuasive contexts. The *Symposium*, written in the first half of the fourth century BCE, seems to include suggestions as to the engagement of doctors in public debates and displays of oratorical skill which the evidence from the oratorical texts of the Hippocratic Collection, dating to the late fifth century BCE, seems to corroborate. There are other hints too from Plato as to the intersection between medicine and new methods of oratorical performance.

In Plato's *Gorgias*, we find Gorgias boasting of his powers of persuasion used in the service of physicians:

> [Gorgias to Socrates] Many times in the past I have visited some patient in the company of my brother and other physicians; when the patient was unwilling to take his medicine, or allow himself to be operated on or cauterized and the doctor could not persuade him, I persuaded him, by no other art than rhetoric.
>
> (Plato, *Gorgias*, 456b1–5)[24]

In this extract, we find Gorgias standing in for the physician, claiming to use his powers of persuasion to have the patient agree to undergo an operation or cauterisation. Given the risks involved in this period of such procedures, Plato's portrayal of Gorgias could imply the manipulative aspect of sophistic speech, a characteristic he would be keen to emphasise given his general hostility to those he labels Sophists and his determination to establish critical distance from them.

There are other points of connection between the doctors and the philosopher Plato. For instance, in *Phaedrus* 270b, Plato has Socrates compare the art of rhetoric with the art of medicine; and in *Theaetetus* 150c, he refers to the philosopher as the midwife of ideas. For the purposes of this book, the connection between medicine and rhetoric is of interest not so much as comparable examples of art (τέχνη), nor insofar as the use of medicine serves as an analogy for philosophical ideas; instead the focus is on the extent to which both medical ideas and oratorical expression are under concurrent development.

This brief sketch indicates some of the evidence for the development of a new mode of writing and expression which defined itself in contrast with verse. Particularly in the case of prose intended for oratorical delivery, we find a self-consciousness about expression and, in some cases, attempts to interweave philosophical issues with expressive experiments, to think through theories in their expression, as it were. Like prose that looks back to verse of earlier periods, oratory in the late fifth-century BCE is rooted in a long-standing tradition; in introducing the background context to this study, it is also necessary to recognise something of the rise of literacy and the changing relationship with oral communication that is a further aspect of the changes that are visible in written expression of the late fifth century BCE. In the final section of this chapter, I note how questions about orality and the nature of oral communication are pertinent to this study of Hippocratic oratory.

The orality of Hippocratic treatises

As already mentioned, the society of the fifth century BCE in the Hellenic world had its roots in oral culture. In the Archaic period in Greece and the surrounding areas, people generally relied on oral rather than written records. The frequently formulaic structure of Homeric epic, including, for instance, repeated set scenes, standard epithets and use of complex ring composition as evidence of oral culture, has been a focus of intense fascination in scholarship, particularly since the work of Milman Parry and Albert Lord in the first half of the twentieth century and their studies of performances of Serbo-Croat poetry as an analogy with the ancient bardic tradition. Cycles of epic poetry were retained in the memory of travelling bards and recited in oral performances from memory; they were the source from which the written versions of the *Iliad* and the *Odyssey* are thought to have been generated, and a form of historical memory for Greek-speaking peoples that pre-dates the emergence of the written historical record (see e.g. Parry 1971 and Lord 1991: 15–48).

The extent to which the Athenian and the wider Hellenic world shifted from being a society largely reliant on oral means of composition, communication and transmission of ideas in the centuries after the Homeric epics were committed to writing, and the implications and nature of this shift, is a wide and multi-layered area of significant debate and discussion. The discussion is such that here I can only touch upon a few works of scholarship that are specific to the question of orality in the Hippocratic Collection and establish their relationship to the aims of this book.

Much work on the orality of the Hippocratic Collection has tended to avoid the evidence of more public and flamboyant oratory, and focused on the notion of oral memory and the question of literacy and its links to epistemology, i.e. how far the use of writing altered ideas and theories of knowledge.[25]

One example of this kind of work is Laurence Totelin's study of the transmission of pharmacological recipes in the Hippocratic Collection – recipes which are concentrated mainly in the gynaecological and nosological treatises (Totelin 2009). Her study builds on the work of scholars such as Lesley Dean-Jones, Iain Lonie and Helen King, who have argued that such recipes offered an insight into the oral tradition of transmission of remedies (Totelin 2009: 3; see Dean-Jones 2003; Lonie 1983; and King 1998: 40–53). In this study, Totelin embraces the notion of an oral tradition operating alongside the written record. She seeks to establish the limits of our evidence in understanding this tradition; cautions against treating the oral and written traditions as separate; and argues that there is a complex relationship between the oral and the written: 'writing is never the exact reflection of spoken language; it transforms the oral word in subtle, yet important ways' (Totelin 2009: 16 and *passim*).

Before Totelin's study, Iain Lonie (1983) considered the extent to which medical practice was modified by literary activity, and whether the Hippocratic writings represent the record in writing of data of a non-literate craft or a new kind of medicine. He considers that Hippocratic 'essays' exemplified by *On Ancient Medicine*, *On the Art*, *On the Nature of Human Beings*, *On Breaths* and *On the Sacred Disease* are not very useful in ascertaining the effects of literacy on medicine because they show features which are common hallmarks of philosophical and sophistic writing of this period but nothing that is specific about the effects of literacy on medicine (Lonie 1983: 148–149) and focuses instead on the presence of categorising and cataloguing features of other Hippocratic texts.[26]

Another antecedent to Totelin's discussion is Lesley Dean-Jones response to Lonie's article and in particular his claim that 'The Greek doctor . . . did not *need* to become literate in order to win professional and social status' (Lonie 1983: 148). In her article on the connection between the rise of literacy and charlatanry in the ancient Greek medical world, Dean-Jones focuses on the first appearance of the criticism of medicine in nonmedical texts in the fourth century BCE, which she claims was also a time when the status of medicine increased 'to that of a *technē* par excellence' (2003: 98). Literacy in the context of Hippocratic medicine, she argues, is linked to changes in the way that doctors were trained and brought about the possibility of access to knowledge and attempts to practice medicine based on book learning that were not possible before literacy (2003: 97–121). This argument leads in a somewhat different direction from the focus of this study, which is the oral qualities of Hippocratic oratory; however, the idea that medical knowledge becomes less exclusive and open to students trained in non-traditional methods is relevant to the nature of Hippocratic oratory. By studying the appearance of oral features of Hippocratic oratory, this study does in a sense put to the test Dean-Jones' use of the term 'charlatan' with its negative connotations and sense of a rupture from pure tradition, and raises questions about the extent to which we can come to firm conclusions about the social status and aims of the authors of Hippocratic oratorical works in a time of unsettled changes.

In contrast to the above-mentioned work on orality, which concentrates on the transmission of medical knowledge or the defence of its status, this study focuses on the orality of performance and public agonistic debate. We find this kind of oral context described in the opening of *On the Nature of Human Beings*, in which the author is decrying deceptive rhetoric and appeals to the crowd as leading people away from the truth:

λέγει δ' αὐτῶν ὁ μέν τις φάσκων ἠέρα εἶναι τοῦτο τὸ ἕν τε καὶ τὸ πᾶν, ὁ δὲ πῦρ, ὁ δὲ ὕδωρ, ὁ δὲ γῆν, καὶ ἐπιλέγει ἕκαστος τῷ ἑωυτοῦ λόγῳ μαρτύριά τε καὶ τεκμήρια ἅ ἐστιν οὐδέν. ὁπότε δὲ γνώμη τῇ αὐτῇ πάντες προσχρέωνται, λέγουσι δ' οὐ ταὐτά, δῆλον ὅτι οὐδὲ γινώσκουσιν. γνοίη δ' ἄν τῷδέ τις μάλιστα παραγενόμενος αὐτοῖσιν ἀντιλέγουσιν· πρὸς γὰρ ἀλλήλους ἀντιλέγοντες οἱ αὐτοὶ ἄνδρες τῶν αὐτῶν ἐναντίον ἀκροατέων οὐδέποτε τρὶς ἐφεξῆς ὁ αὐτὸς περιγίνεται ἐν τῷ λόγῳ, ἀλλὰ ποτὲ μὲν οὗτος ἐπικρατεῖ, τοτὲ δὲ οὗτος, τοτὲ δὲ ᾧ ἂν τύχῃ μάλιστα ἡ γλῶσσα ἐπιρρυεῖσα πρὸς τὸν ὄχλον.

They argue about this thing one saying that the air is the one and all another fire, another water, another earth, and each selects for their argument testimony and evidence, which are worth nothing. So when they all speak the same ideas, but say different things, it is clear that they do not understand these things. One can realise these things especially when being beside them arguing: for the same men are never opposed to the others. In victory three times in a row in a discussion but once one prevails with an argument than another then whoever has chance to have the most fluid tongue before the crowd.

(*On the Nature of Human Beings*, 1.1)

The competitive and showy nature of these debates is also indicated here, with some suggestion as to their spontaneous and improvised qualities and to the importance of impressive language in the reference to 'ἡ γλῶσσα ἐπιρρυεῖσα' 'fluent tongue'.

Within the Hippocratic Collection, there is clear evidence that a significant proportion of the treatises were designed for this kind of delivery context, as speeches which were intended to make an aesthetic as well as theoretical impression. Rosalind Thomas' work on literacy and orality, particularly in natural philosophy and historiography, is an important landmark in discussions about orality which is closely related to the aspects of orality that this study aims to engage with.[27] In particular, Thomas' work in *Herodotus in Context* (2000) on Herodotus' engagement in public debate of topics of natural philosophy is an important precedent for this study – though the focus here is from the point of view of the Hippocratic Collection rather than Herodotus' *Histories*. As Thomas does with Herodotus' writing, this study will analyse the way in which Hippocratic authors ostensibly contributing to public debates seek to persuade and convince their audience. Thomas' work on *epideixis* in relation to the Hippocratic oratorical treatises will be discussed further below, in Chapter 3.

Finally, it is important to mention Jouanna's analysis of the rhetoric of the Hippocratic Collection in an article published in 1984 – 'Rhetoric and Medicine in the Hippocratic Collection: contribution to the history of rhetoric in the fifth century' – which is an initial landmark in the emerging discussions of the orality of Hippocratic performance oratory and which provides some justification for the focus of this book.[28]

In the article, Jouanna outlines evidence for the existence of a group of treatises within the Hippocratic Collection which should be considered 'oral' in the sense that they contain signs that they were composed for the purposes of speech-making. Jouanna claims that a distinction between treatises composed for publication as written documents and those composed for the purposes of oral dissemination can be established. This distinction depends on the presence or absence of words that indicate whether a given treatise is likely to have been delivered orally or written down. He analyses the presence or absence of γράφειν and λέγειν and related words in the treatises, noting: 'If we add up the uses of φημί, ἐρέω, λέγω [verbs which can all mean 'to say'], leaving to one side ambiguous case of *Eight Month's Child*, there are 76 uses in 'oral' works as against 23 for the all the rest of the Hippocratic Collection' (Jouanna 1984: 32, n.1).[29] The distinction between oral and written treatises, then, is not cut and dried, but clear enough for a certain group of treatises to be considered 'oral'.[30]

This is a useful, if not entirely reliable, analysis. The presence of verbs referring to speaking is a strong indicator of the close relationship of any given Hippocratic treatise to the context of oral dissemination; there is always the possibility, however, that authors of treatises delivered their works as speeches and then wrote them up for a reading audience, with references to writing rather than speaking; and *vice versa* that references to speaking can be understood as ways to enliven a text that was never in fact delivered in speech before a live audience. Nevertheless, Jouanna's work does provide the basis for further discussion of what a Hippocratic oratorical treatise is, and what it seeks to achieve persuasively.

In the above, then, we have seen that among the scholarship on the increasing move away from oral to written communication in the fifth century BCE in Greece, there are several important precedents for the study of the oral features of Hippocratic oratory on which this study seeks to build. Further discussion of what these features are and why they might be employed can be found below, particularly in Chapters 3 and 4. Overall, the topic of the orality of Hippocratic treatises has begun to be investigated, but this is a complex subject which requires further investigation, and in which different aspects of the Collection invite different approaches and questions.

With the five examples of Hippocratic oratorical treatises selected for this study specifically in mind, we have seen in the introduction above how they fit into a tradition of public debate on medical topics for which there are significant Pre-Socratic, Sophistic and historiographic models; we have also seen how as far as Hippocratic oratorical texts are concerned, there is a tendency for self-conscious manipulation of and experimentation with expression which runs concurrently with the explanation and exposition of new medical theories; that this is a phenomenon which we also find reflected in specific Pre-Socratic and Sophistic texts is a point worth considering further and which warrants investigation and close analysis of persuasive strategies employed.

In the next chapter, I consider in more detail the notion of an overlap between thought processes and expression and explore specific examples of models for the kind of persuasive patterning that is characteristic of Hippocratic expository prose.

Notes

1 See my discussion of 'oral' treatises in the Collection and of Jouanna's 1984 article below.
2 See, for instance, Chang (2005) on the range of locations referred to in the Collection.
3 'La Collection hippocratique n'existe d'une manière authentique que depuis le temps d'Hérophile et de ses élèves' (Littré 1973 [1827]: 263). See also Jouanna and Magdelaine (1999: 8–20), Nutton (2013 [2004]: 53–62), Smith (1979). See Craik (2015) for an up-to-date overview of the contents of the collection along with detailed records of editions and comments on context and dates of the treatises. See also Jouanna (1999) as the standard introductory historical synthesis on the Hippocratic Collection and Sigerist (1951–1961) with a broader historical narrative overview of ancient Greek medicine.
4 Pinault (1992), Smith (1990).
5 The main ancient references to the historical Hippocrates are: Plato, *Protagoras* 311b-c, *Phaedrus* 270c-d; Aristotle, *Politics* 7.1326a.14–16. See Smith (1979: 31–43) for an overview of discussions regarding the Hippocratic question and a further contribution to this strand of scholarship.

6   For an exploration of some philosophical aspects of the treatises in the collection, see for example van der Eijk (2005) and Hankinson (1991); for an example of an analysis of links between history writing and Hippocratic texts see Jouanna (2005); see Thomas (2000: 42–68) for an example of an exploration of the relationship between ethnography of health in Herodotus' *Histories* and in the Hippocratic writings.

7   Jones (1923: vol. 1: xxiv), notes that '[A] most important group of works consists of those in which the philosophic element predominates over the scientific, the writers being anxious, not to advance the practice of medicine, but to bring medicine under the control of philosophic dogma'. A good example of a Hippocratic treatise that contains different kinds of material in separate parts of the treatise is *Airs, Waters, Places*, which Bottin (1986: 9), notes contains different levels of discussion: medical, ethnographic and ecological.

8   One striking and famous example is Homer's *Iliad*, I, 1–187, where Apollo is described as having brought a plague upon the Greek army. See further, for example, Holmes (2010) on the historical development of the concept of the body, the soul and the person, focusing on the Hippocratic Collection as central to this development.

9   Laskaris (2002) and Mann (2012) are notable and important exceptions.

10 'Ni la forme sophistique du discours, ni les rencontres avec les théories de Diogène d'Apollonie ou d'Empédocle ne doivent masquer une réalité plus profonde: le traité plonge ses racines dans la médecine hippocratique au sens large du terme. On y a vu à tort un discours de sophiste égaré dans la *Collection hippocratique*. Par le ton, par les thèmes généraux sur l'art, par le détail des explications physiologiques, l'œuvre est en accord avec le fonds commun de la médecine hippocratique.'

11 'Le traité de l'*Art* présente des analogies dans la forme avec celui des *Vents*. C'est également un discours épidictique composé avec la technique sophistique par un médecin qui démontre une thèse. Mais la thèse est fort différente: alors que l'auteur des *Vents* soutient que l'air est la cause de toutes les maladies, l'auteur de l'*Art* montre que la médecine existe en tant que τέχνη, en tant qu'« art ».'

12 For overviews of the development of rhetoric in ancient Greece, see for example Kennedy (1963) and Cole (1991), the latter arguing that rhetoric is a largely Platonic and Aristotelian invention. On the development of oratory see for example Habinek (2005), Gagarin (2002), Grethlein (2013) and Worthington (2007). See also Adrados (2005: 161–174) for a linguistic perspective on the development of 'scientific' language.

13 Parmenides, active around the end of the sixth and beginning of the fifth century BCE, is another important predecessor of Hippocratic oratory. Like Empedocles, he is a natural philosopher writing in verse associated with medicine: an inscription found on a herm in Velia in Italy suggests that Parmenides was linked with the study of medicine. See Ebner (1962), and Greco and Krinzinger (1994). See Chapter 2 for further discussion of Parmenides' work as a model for Hippocratic oratory.

14 'nam primus post eos quos poetae tradiderunt movisse aliqua circa rhetoricen Empedocles dicitur. artium autem scriptores antiquissimi Corax et Tisias Siculi, quos insecutus est vir eiusdem insulae Gorgias Leontinus, Empedoclis, ut traditur, discipulus' (3.1.8).

15 Lucretius was clearly strongly influenced in places by early Greek prose writing: see, for instance, Segal (1970) on close connections between descriptions of seizure in *On the Nature of Things* and *On Breaths*.

16 There is an extensive secondary literature on the shift from poetic to new forms of authoritative expression. Most useful for the purposes of this project is Most (1999) on the poetics of early Greek Philosophy and Thomas (1992); see also Kennedy (1963, 1994) for a standard introductory survey of the development of 'rhetoric' in ancient Greece and Cole (1991) for a key challenge to the standard narrative; these works contain essential further bibliography on their respective areas of enquiry.

17 Craik (1998: 33) notes that the Hippocratic treatises *On Places in the Human Being* may be the earliest work of the Hippocratic Collection and one of the earliest works of Greek prose.

18 Thucydides *On the Peloponnesian War*, 2.47–55. See for example Dawson and Harvey (1986) on Herodotus as a medical writer. On historiography and fifth-century enquiries into nature see especially Lateiner (1986), Thomas (2006; 2000: 168–212).

19 I would contest, however, Goldhill's main conclusion in the *Invention of Prose* which separates prose into distinct areas – historical prose, rhetoric, philosophy, the prose of medical science: 'Where historical prose found authority in the critical evaluated narrative of events, where rhetoric found authority in persuasive performance, philosophy seeks to place authority in the power of argument itself, and the prose of medical science rests its authority on the power of description to make the world comprehensible' (Goldhill 2002: 110).As will be argued later in this book, the division between different genres of prose is only useful up to a point: in fact, the evidence from the Hippocratic 'oral' treatises is that medical prose, to take one of these categories, combines all of the features noted: critical evaluated narrative of events, persuasive performance, the power of argument, as well as on the power of description.

20 See also Richard Buxton's study of persuasion in ancient Greek tragedy, which highlights the sociological aspect of this shift from verse to prose arguing that prior to the rise of the democratic state, debates about stately affairs were closed off from the public and held only between those who were *already* in power (1982: 5–27).

21 On Gorgias and rhetoric *as* philosophy, see for example Wardy (2009).

22 See Kerferd (1981) for a standard overview of the rise of the Sophists.

23 'δηλοῖ δὲ τοῦτο Γοργίας τε ὁ Λεοντῖνος ἐν πολλοῖς πάνυ φορτικήν τε καὶ ὑπέρογκον ποιῶν τὴν κατασκευὴν καὶ "οὐ πόρρω διθυράμβων τινῶν" ἔνια φθεγγόμενος, καὶ τῶν ἐκείνου συνουσιαστῶν οἱ περὶ Λικύμνιον καὶ Πῶλον. ἥψατο δὲ καὶ τῶν Ἀθήνησι ῥητόρων ἡ ποιητική τε καὶ τροπικὴ φράσις, ὡς μὲν Τίμαιός φησι, Γοργίου ἄρξαντος ἡνίκ᾽Ἀθήναζε πρεσβεύων κατεπλήξατο τοὺς ἀκούοντας τῆι δημηγορίαι.'

24 'πολλάκις γὰρ ἤδη ἔγωγεμετὰ τοῦ ἀδελφοῦ καὶ μετὰ τῶν ἄλλων ἰατρῶν εἰσελθὼνπαρά τινα τῶν καμνόντων οὐχὶ ἐθέλοντα ἢ φάρμακον πιεῖν ἢτεμεῖν ἢ καῦσαι παρασχεῖν τῷ ἰατρῷ, οὐ δυναμένού τοῦἰατροῦ πεῖσαι, ἐγὼ ἔπεισα, οὐκ ἄλλῃ τέχνῃ ἢ τῇ ῥητορικῇ.'

25 See e.g. Kudlein (1967). On links between literacy and epistemology in medical contexts see Pigeaud (1988), Miller (1990).

26 See also, e.g. Kollesch (1992) for discussion of the notion of orality in a Hippocratic context.

27 See Thomas (1992: 101–127) for a discussion of some of the central issues surrounding the topic of oral communication in early Greece that bear upon any interpretation of ancient texts; see also Thomas (2003: 163–188) for a discussion of the relationship between prose text and its performance and the issue of authority

in choice of medium for communicating ideas. Other recent work on orality in ancient Greece include Watson (2001), Nagy (2002), Cooper (2007).

28 The title of the article in French is 'Rhétorique et Médecine dans la collection Hippocratique: contribution à l'histoire de la rhétorique au Ve siècle'.

29 'Si l'on fait le total des emplois de φημί, ἐρέω, λέγω, en laissant de côté le cas ambigu du *Fœtus de huit mois*, on arrive à 76 emplois pour les oeuvres orales contre 23 pour tout le reste de la Collection hippocratique.'

30 This group consists of (in alphabetical order): *Airs, Waters, Places; Diseases IV; Diseases of Women; On Ancient Medicine; On Breaths; On the Art; On the Eight Month's Foetus; On the Nature of the Child; On the Nature of Human Beings; On the Sacred Disease; Regimen I; On the Heart; Regimen in Acute Diseases.*

References

Adrados, F. R. (2005), *A History of the Greek Language*: *From Its Origins to the Present*. Leiden: Brill.

Bottin, L. (ed. and trans.) (1986), *Ippocrate. Arie Acque Luoghi*. Venezia: Marsilio Editori.

Buxton, R. G. A. (1982), *Persuasion in Greek Tragedy: A Study of Peitho*. Cambridge: Cambridge University Press. 5–27.

Chang, H. (2005), 'The Cities of the Hippocratic Doctors' in van der Eijk, Ph. J. (ed.), *Hippocrates in Context. Papers Read at the XIth International Hippocrates Colloquium. University of Newcastle upon Tyne, 27–31 August 2002*. Studies in Ancient Medicine 31. Leiden: Brill. 157–171.

Cole, T. (1991), *The Origins of Rhetoric in Ancient Greece*. Baltimore, MD; London: The John Hopkins University Press.

Cooper, C. (ed.) (2007), *Politics of Orality*. Leiden; Boston, MA: Brill.

Craik, E. M. (2015), *The 'Hippocratic' Corpus: Content and Context*. London: Routledge.

Craik, E. M. (ed. and trans.) (1998), *Hippocrates: Places in Man*. Oxford: Clarendon Press.

Dawson, W. R. and Harvey, F. D. (1986), 'Herodotus as a Medical Writer' in *Bulletin of the Institute of Classical Studies*. Oxford: Blackwell. 33: 87–96.

Dean-Jones, L. (2003), 'Literacy and the Charlatan in Ancient Greek Medicine' in Yunis, H. (ed.), *Written Texts and the Rise of Literate Culture in Ancient Greece*. Cambridge: Cambridge University Press. 97–121.

Ebner, P. (1962), 'Scuole di medicina a Velia e a Salerno.' *Apollo: Bolletino dei Musei Provinciali del Salernitano*. Salerno: Mondadori Electa. 2: 125–136.

van der Eijk, Ph. J. (ed.) (2005), *Medicine and Philosophy in Classical Antiquity: Doctors and Philosophers on Nature, Soul, Health and Disease*. Cambridge; New York: Cambridge University Press.

Gagarin, M. (2002), *Antiphon the Athenian: Oratory, Law, and Justice in the Age of the Sophists*. Austin, TX: University of Texas Press.

Goldhill, S. (2002), *The Invention of Prose*. Greece & Rome New Surveys in the Classics, No. 32. Oxford: Oxford University Press.

Greco, G. and F. Krinzinger (eds.) (1994), *Velia: Studi e Ricerche*. Modena: Panini.

Grethlein, J. (2013), 'Democracy, Oratory, and the Rise of Historiography in Fifth-century Greece' in Arnason, J. P. *et al.* (eds.), *The Greek Polis and the Invention of Democracy: A Politico-cultural Transformation and Its Interpretations.* Chichester, West Sussex: Wiley Blackwell.

Habinek, T. (2005), *Ancient Rhetoric and Oratory.* Malden, MA; Oxford: Blackwell Publications.

Hankinson, R. J. (1991), 'Greek Medical Models of Mind' in Everson, S. (ed.), *Psychology.* Cambridge; New York: Cambridge University Press. 194–217.

Holmes, B. (2010), *The Symptom and the Subject: The Emergence of the Physical Body in Ancient Greece.* Princeton, NJ; Oxford: Princeton University Press.

Jones, W. H. S. (ed. and trans.) (1923), *Hippocrates II.* [reprinted 1998–2005]. Loeb Classical Library 148. Cambridge, MA; London: Harvard University Press.

Jouanna, J. (2005), 'Cause and Crisis in Historians and Medical Writers of the Classical Period' in *Hippocrates in Context: Papers Read at the XIth International Hippocrates Colloquium (University of Newcastle upon Tyne, 27–31 August 2002).* Leiden: Brill. 3–28.

Jouanna, J. (ed. and trans.) (2002 [1975]), *Corpus Medicorum Graecorum* I, 1, 3. *Hippocrate. La nature de l'homme.* Berlin: Akademie-Verlag.

Jouanna, J. (1999), *Hippocrates.* Baltimore, MD; London: Johns Hopkins University Press.

Jouanna, J. (ed. and trans.) (1988), *Hippocrate. Tome V, 1re partie. Des vents; De l'art.* Paris: Les Belles Lettres.

Jouanna, J. (1984), 'Rhétorique et médecine dans la collection Hippocratique: contribution à l'histoire de la rhétorique au Ve siècle.' *Revue des Études greques 97.* Paris: Les Belles Lettres. 26–44.

Jouanna, J. and Magdelaine, C. (eds. and trans.) (1999), *L'art de la médecine: serment, ancienne médecine, art, airs, eaux, lieux, maladie sacrée, nature de l'homme, pronostic, aphorismes.* Paris: Flammarion.

Kerferd, G. (1981), *The Sophistic Movement.* Cambridge; New York: Cambridge University Press.

Kennedy, G. A. (1994), *A New History of Classical Rhetoric.* Princeton, NJ: Princeton University Press.

Kennedy, G. A. (1963), *The Art of Persuasion in Ancient Greece.* Princeton, NJ: Princeton University Press.

King, H. (1998), *Hippocrates' Woman: Reading the Female Body in Ancient Greece.* London: Routledge.

Kollesch, J. (1992), 'Zur Mündlichkeit hippokratischer Schriften' in López Férez, J. A. (ed.), *Tratados hipocráticos (Estudios acerca de su contenido, forma e influencia).* Madrid: Universidad Nacional de Educacion a Distancia. 335–342.

Kudlein, F. (1967), *Der Beginn des medizinischen Denkens bei den Griechen.* Zürich; Stuttgart: Artemis Verlag.

Kurke, L. (2011), *Aesopic Conversations: Popular Tradition, Cultural Dialogue, and the Invention of Greek Prose.* Princeton, NJ; Oxford: Princeton University Press.

Laskaris, J. (2002), *The Art is Long: On the Sacred Disease and the Scientific Tradition.* Leiden; Boston, MA: Brill.

Lateiner, D. (1986), 'The Empirical Element in the Methods of Early Greek Medical Writers and Herodotus: A Shared Epistemological Response' in *Antichthon*. Cambridge: Cambridge University Press. 20: 1–20.

Littré, É. (ed. and trans.) (1973-1989 [1839-1861]), *Œuvres complètes d'Hippocrate*. Amsterdam: Adolf M. Hakkert. Reprint of Paris: J.B. Baillière, 1839–1861.

Lonie, I. M. (1983), 'Literacy and the Development of Hippocratic Medicine' in Lassere, F. and Mudry, Ph. (eds.), *Formes de pensée dans la collection hippocratique: actes du IVe Colloque international hippocratique*. Genève: Droz. 145–161.

Lord, A. B. (1991), *Epic Singers and Oral Tradition*. New York; London: Cornell University Press.

Mann, J. E. (2012), *Hippocrates, On the Art of Medicine*. Leiden; Boston, MA: Brill.

Miller, G. L. (1990), 'Literacy and the Hippocratic Art: Reading, Writing and Epistemology in Ancient Greek Medicine.' *Journal of the History of Medicine and Allied Sciences*. Oxford: Oxford University Press. 45: 11–40.

Most, G. W. (1999), 'The Poetics of Early Greek Philosophy' in Long, A. A. (ed.), *The Cambridge Companion to Early Greek Philosophy*. Cambridge: Cambridge University Press. 332–362.

Nagy, G. (2002), *Plato's Rhapsody and Homer's Music: The Poetics of the Panathenaic Festival in Classical Athens* Washington, DC: Center for Hellenic Studies, Trustees for Harvard University; Athens, Greece: Foundation of the Hellenic World; Cambridge, MA; London: Distributed by Harvard University Press.

Nutton, V. (2013 [2004]), *Ancient Medicine*. London: Routledge.

Parry, A. (ed.) (1971), *The Making of Homeric Verse: The Collected Papers of Milman Parry*. Oxford: Clarendon Press.

Pigeaud, J. (1988), 'Le style d'Hippocrate ou l'écriture fondatrice de la médecine' in Detienne, M. (ed.), *Les savoirs de l'écriture en Grèce ancienne*. Villeneuve-d'Ascq, France: Presses universitaires de Lille. 305–329.

Pinault, J. (ed. and trans.) (1992), *Hippocratic Lives and Legends*. Leiden; New York; Köln: Brill.

Segal, C. (1970), 'Lucretius, Epilepsy and the Hippocratic *On Breaths*.' in *Classical Philology* 65 (3). The University of Chicago Press, 180–182.

Sigerist, H. E. (1951–1961), *A History of Medicine*. 2 Vols. New York: Oxford University Press.

Smith, W. D. (1979), *The Hippocratic Tradition*. Ithaca, New York: Cornell University Press.

Smith, W. (ed. and trans.) (1990), *Pseudepigraphic Writings*. Leiden; New York; Köln: Brill.

Thomas, R. (2006), 'The Intellectual Milieu of Herodotus' in C. Dewald, J. Marincola (eds.), *The Cambridge Companion to Herodotus*. Cambridge: Cambridge University Press. 60–75.

Thomas, R. (2003), 'Prose Performance Texts' in Yunis, H. (ed.), *Written Texts and the Rise of Literate Culture in Ancient Greece*. Cambridge: Cambridge University Press. 163–188.

Thomas, R. (2000), *Herodotus in Context: Ethnography, Science and the Art of Persuasion*. Cambridge: Cambridge University Press.

Thomas, R. (1992), *Literacy and Orality in Ancient Greece*. Cambridge: Cambridge University Press. 101–127.

Totelin, L. (2009), *Hippocratic Recipes: Oral and Written Transmission of Pharmacological Knowledge in Fifth- and Fourth-Century Greece*. Leiden; Boston, MA: Brill.

Wardy, R. (2009), 'The Philosophy of Rhetoric and the Rhetoric of Philosophy' in Gunderson, E. (ed.), *The Cambridge Companion to Ancient Rhetoric*. Cambridge: Cambridge University Press. 43–58.

Watson, J. (ed.) (2001), *Speaking Volumes: Orality and Literacy in the Greek and Roman World*. Leiden; Boston, MA: Brill.

Worthington, I. (ed.) (2007), *A Companion to Greek Rhetoric*. Malden, MA: Oxford: Blackwell Publications.

2 Models of *logos* and medical oratory

We saw in the first chapter how Hippocratic oratorical texts seem to emerge from a tradition of public declamation on topics associated with natural philosophy and that there are specific precursors for Hippocratic oratory among Pre-Socratic thinkers. We also saw how, like Pre-Socratic thinkers, Hippocratic performance prose is subject to the push and pull of underlying shifts which characterise the development of prose expression in the fifth century BCE in Greece, namely the move towards ever-greater reliance on and respect for the written over the spoken word and the move away from verse form as the main mode of authoritative communication.

Another way of framing and encapsulating the shift from verse to prose, from oral to literate, and of thinking more deeply about the nature of the emergence of different ways of thinking, is through the notion of an emergence of a new kind of *logos*. The term *logos* is fraught with complexity and can mean anything from story to account to logical analysis; it can encompass content and form of thought, as well communication context, and as such has sometimes been contrasted with the term *muthos*, associated with mythic modes of thought and expression, in studies seeking to analyse the changes in thinking taking place in the fifth century BCE.

Before considering the notions of *muthos* and *logos* further, it is useful to establish a common modern definition of logical argument. The following is found in *The Cambridge Dictionary of Philosophy*:

> Argument . . . [is] a sequence of statements such that some of them (the premises) purport to give reason to accept another of them (the conclusion). Since we speak of bad arguments and weak arguments, the premises of an argument need not really support the conclusion, but they must give some appearance of doing so or the term 'argument' is misapplied.
>
> (Purtill 1995: 37)

Argument is essentially a certain relationship that holds between sequences of statements; this informs modern understanding – in academic writing, at least – of valid explanation.

Stories and myths, for example, can have 'arguments' in the sense that they can be constructed around plots that must contain some kind of internal 'logic': there must be reasons or causes for the developments that take place within the narrative. The difference between the 'argument' of a narrative and the 'argument' of a series of assertions is that the latter claims that the connection between one statement and the next is *necessary*. Stories and myths may contradict one another by offering different versions of the statements that they make but they generally do not set out to contradict one another *incontrovertibly*.[1] Stories and myths may therefore offer explanations, but not – in modern academic terms – valid explanations.

The first explicit formal analysis of the notion of valid and invalid explanation is found famously in Aristotle's fourth-century *Prior Analytics*. It is the contention of this study that in the centuries preceding Aristotle's famous account, we cannot assume that a notion of argument resembling the example given above was standard or readily available, or even that there existed a pre-established model of argument; this point has implications for what might have seemed convincing to a fifth-century audience.

In this chapter, I consider firstly the notion of *logos* in relation to the selected five Hippocratic treatises. I demonstrate how, although some Hippocratic treatises have been read through a lens of philosophically robust and rigid criteria of argument – readings which follow broadly in Aristotle's tradition – Hippocratic texts convey meaning at different levels and in different manners from the philosophically strict notion of argument. Against this kind of reading, I set notions of *logos* that are pre-rational and relate to realms of meaning beyond the written word and operate more loosely and associatively rather than by rigid criteria. I argue that for too long, rigid readings of Hippocratic texts have prevailed, and that the associative meanings they convey have been downplayed or dismissed as trivial.

In the second section of the chapter, I explore scholarship on the relationship between style and thought, arguing that here too a black-and-white approach to notions of form and content has prevailed, with much work produced that assumes to varying degrees that style is superfluous to content, and that a neat division between form and content is in fact possible. I highlight the way in which aesthetic assumptions about what a 'classical' work should look like lie buried within some recent readings of early Greek prose, and identify the ways in which such an approach is limited. I also identify works of scholarship that attempt to analyse the complexity of prose writing head on, aware of and sensitive to preconceptions about what makes a text persuasive and what qualifies as good argument.

Finally, in the third section of this chapter, I explore models of explanation in early Greek prose. The idea here is to gain some sense of the precedents which were available to the Hippocratic authors for making a case to an audience. Examining specific connections between Parmenides', Heraclitus' and Herodotus' work and passages from the author of the Hippocratic treatise *On Breaths*, this third section of the chapter demonstrates the presence of a heady mix of truth claims, patterning in phrasing and expression and underlying notions of how 'truth' must appear in the Hippocratic work, and a genealogical connection with the work of this author's predecessors.

Logos and rational argument in Hippocratic oratory

In discussions of ancient philosophical texts, there exists a sizeable and intricate body of scholarship on the development of logic. A key example from this, relevant to discussion of Hippocratic oratory, is R. J. Hankinson's study *Cause and Explanation in Ancient Greek Thought*.

I turn now to Hankinson's comments on the Hippocratic treatise *On the Sacred Disease*, to illustrate one way in which Hippocratic explanation has been shown to exhibit the hallmarks of logical argument along the lines of the definition cited above in *The Cambridge Dictionary of Philosophy*. After this, I discuss the work of scholars who identify other modes of 'logic' in early Greek writing which complicate the picture that Hankinson paints of the linear development of 'logical thinking' from mythic or superstitious modes of thought in natural philosophical texts.

Hankinson's aim in his study is to consider 'what sort of thing . . . the Greeks [thought] causes were, and how . . . they [conceived] of adequacy in explanation' (Hankinson 1998: 1). He focuses on the Hippocratic treatise *On the Sacred Disease* and argues that in this treatise 'The old methods and prescriptions of the temple doctors (the wearing of magic amulets, divination on the basis of dreams experienced while sleeping in sacred sanctuaries, prayer) were challenged by a new, rational medical paradigm' (Hankinson 1998: 51). He identifies *On the Sacred Disease* as an example of a new rational paradigm in thinking, and is a standard-bearer for an approach to the Hippocratic Collection that emphasises its rational qualities as evidence of the earliest progression towards the development of modern scientific method.[2]

The new, rational medical paradigm Hankinson argues is apparent in *On the Sacred Disease* is said to be an 'allopathic principle' (i.e. that opposites cure opposites), a paradigm that is found throughout the Hippocratic Collection. In the line

φύσιν δὲ ἕκαστον ἔχει καὶ δύναμιν εφ᾽ ἑωτοῦ, καὶ οὐδὲν ἄπορόν ἐστιν οὐδ᾽ ἀμήχανον

Each [thing / element] has a nature and power of its own and none is hopeless or incapable of treatment

(*On the Sacred Disease*, 18.1)

Hankinson finds an allopathic principle that is intended to regulate treatment, and which is related to the general causal principle:

> For any x, and y, and any F, if x is the cause of y's being F, then removal of x will contribute to the suppression of F.
>
> (Hankinson 1998: 53)

Hankinson goes on to claim that it is this causal principle that is at the core of the author's belief that the 'sacred disease' can be explained and treated in terms of nature and that this same basic principle is at the root of the author's rejection of the prescriptions of the magico-religious healers.

The general causal principle that Hankinson uncovers here is also applicable to the cause of the sacred disease that is given. The author of *On the Sacred Disease* states, for example, that an excessive down-flow of phlegm from the brain is the primary cause of seizure in a patient. In Hankinson's terms, excessive phlegm in the veins (x) is the main cause of the body (y) being prone to episodes of the 'sacred' disease (F). The idea that 'removal of x will contribute to the suppression of F' is consistent with the idea stated in the treatise that the dissipation of the phlegm leads to the symptoms passing away

Against Hankinson's analysis, we can set studies into the 'logic' of mythic modes of thought. A mainstay of such scholarship is Marcel Detienne's *The Masters of the Truth in Archaic Greece* (1996), itself grounded in structuralism and the work of scholars such as Jean-Pierre Vernant (1983). Detienne's and Vernant's studies explore the idea of the 'logic of myth' as an ancestor of 'rational logic'. Detienne's enquiry into the pre-rational nature of 'truth' and the birth of the scientific notion of truth (in a loose sense, associated with objectivity, communicability, and unity) offers a counterpoint to Hankinson's identification of the development of rational argument in the Hippocratic Collection.

Hankinson's study broadly aims to identify positive contributions in a movement towards a philosophically robust notion of 'rationality'. By contrast, Detienne seeks to identify a variety of levels of logic operating within the same text.

In discussing the first example of extended argument in Greece, Parmenides' poem on the journey towards truth, Detienne notes that

> When Alētheia appeared in the prelude to Parmenides' poem, it did not spring, fully developed, from the philosopher's brain . . . [the] mythical and religious imagery [we find in the poem] is singularly at odds with abstract philosophical thought focusing, for example, on Being itself. All these features, whose religious character is undeniable, definitely point us toward certain philosophico-religious circles in which a philosopher was still just a wise man, even a magus.
>
> (Detienne 1996: 37)

Detienne's aim in his study is in one sense to write a pre-history of Parmenides' poem analysing, from a largely anthropological perspective, the processes by which the 'truth' (Alētheia) of mythical and magico-religious speech in Archaic Greece – which is not opposed to falsehood, but is rather entwined in a relationship with oblivion (*Lethe*) – was deliberately abandoned and gives way to the secular, communal, and contestable notion of 'truth' that is broadly familiar to us in the early scientific tradition.[3] From the point of view of the development of argument, Detienne is examining and charting the movement away from the ambiguity of organisational structures of myth to the explicit principle of contradiction that develops with rational argument, as understood in Hankinson's terms.

Detienne argues that

> The poet's speech never solicits agreement from its listeners or assent from a social group, no more than does a king of justice: it is deployed with all the majesty of oracular speech. It does not attempt to establish a chain of words in real time that would gather force from human approval or disagreement. To the extent that magico-religious speech transcends human time, it also transcends human beings. It is not the manifestation of an individual's will or thought, nor does it constitute the expression of any particular agent or individual. It is the attribute and privilege of a social function.
>
> (Detienne 1996: 75)

In magico-religious speech of the archaic period, according to Detienne, there is no possibility of contradiction because such speech does not seek consent from others and is bound within a social function that assures its status; it transcends, or seeks to transcend, the boundaries of human communication.

The transition from magico-religious speech to rational dialogue is described in Detienne's study; it is a complex transition that is said to develop along two main strands. The first is through Sophistic speech which is said to inhabit the sphere of opinion and which 'was certainly an instrument, but not a way to know reality. *Logos* was a reality in itself, but not a signifier pointing to the signified. In this type of speech there was no distance between words and things' (Detienne 1996: 118). This idea of words embodying a reality is one that I will explore further in Chapter 4 below. The second is through philosophical reflection in which the correspondence between language and reality was under scrutiny (Detienne 1996: 106)

Although Detienne's work is focused partly on a period well before that of the Hippocratic treatises and in its establishment of architectural 'models' of magico-religous and secular speech the study often makes use of neat dichotomies that may or may not stand up to further historical investigation, it offers a useful counterpoint to studies that emphasise the 'rationality' of early science over its 'pre-rational' history, such as Hankinson's.[4]

Hankinson's analysis of the *On the Sacred Disease* is problematic in that it neatens up the edges of the ideas presented and avoids considering the significance of the inconsistencies in favour of singling out whatever is judged to be consistent, or universal. There are many other details of the description of the cause of the 'sacred' disease that would not fit with Hankinson's causal principle: for example, the fact that the symptoms sometimes occur on the left- and sometimes on the right-hand side of the body, and the idea that the root cause of excessive phlegm in the brain is hereditary and the reason air being cut off causes seizure is said to be that air needs to move around constantly. Such factors do not come under the 'causal principle' that Hankinson outlines, yet it is not clear whether the author sees them as highly significant components of his account or not.

Hankinson notes that

> Sacred Disease recalls Pre-Socratic naturalism in its pretensions to explain (and indeed control) physical phenomena on the basis of an abstract and general causal theory, yet one which seems none the less wholly to outrun its evidential base. Although it is loosely based upon observations, and while it is designed to account for certain facts which the sacred theory [of the magico-religious healers] cannot (such as its heritability, and the fact that it affects young people to a disproportionate extent), the profane, rational account is itself mumbo-jumbo. The avowed method of seeking causally relevant conjunctions of general facts is poorly prosecuted in practice, and in many cases it is unclear if the alleged phenomena upon which the theory is based could ever have been observed, much less that they support the author's own physical hypotheses at the expense of any others.
>
> (Hankinson 1998: 54)

It is clear that the author does not share with us a notion of the overwhelming *primacy* of an 'evidential base' or of the valid prosecution of arguments. So, to judge the treatise as 'poorly prosecuted' is to apply very different standards of argument to the treatise from those that the author apparently has in mind.

The persuasive function of *On the Sacred Disease*, then, includes the expression of oppositional thinking – to take one aspect of his work that is mentioned here – at different levels in his writing and this must be taken into account as part of the author's explanatory resources: that is, we must consider why we find opposites described in the make-up and functioning of the body concurrently with oppositional phrasing in the language of the treatise as well as oppositional positioning between the author and his opponents and the connection between these. The 'allopathic principle' is not only more than a notion of healing but also *not* a principle so much as a characteristic pattern of thought. This is not to deny the presence of remarkable advances in reasoning that we can witness in this treatise, but to acknowledge the complexity of the context in which they are expressed.

There are many examples of Hippocratic oratory displaying something of the notion that *logos* is a reality in itself. In *On the Sacred Disease*, for example, the rejection of the magico-religious healers' arguments shows an obvious engagement with magico-religious modes of thinking (we may not be able to reconstruct these fully, but the account given by the author for the purposes of criticism may give us some idea) (*On the Sacred Disease* 1.1–13). The author's own theological point of view is also an important feature of the treatise.[5] Similarly, the references to the operation of climatic and heavenly phenomena in both treatises echo mythical accounts because they are not subject to argument, whereas other claims in the treatise are. The discussion of opposing winds in *On the Sacred Disease* seems, as Julie Laskaris has pointed out, of a different order to other claims in the treatise about the triggering causes of the disease.[6] In *On Breaths*, the claims that 'air is the basis for all things' and that it has power over heavenly bodies are mythico-religious in tone (*On Breaths* 3.1–3).

This book seeks, then, loosely following authors such as Detienne and Vernant – insofar as they attempt to unravel the 'logic' of ambiguous modes of expression – to detect some of the underlying patterns in persuasive language used in Hippocratic oratorical texts that fail to meet commonly applied notions of valid argument and scientific method and that contrast with the presence of examples of rational argumentation as defined by Hankinson.

Another scholar who has sought to shed light on the processes by which a shift from *muthos* to *logos* in explanatory prose writing occurred in ancient Greece is Geoffrey Lloyd. His studies contain much research that was groundbreaking when first published and remains a standard point of reference for any further work in this field. *Polarity and Analogy: Two Types of Argumentation in Early Greek Thought* (1966), *Magic, Reason and Experience* (1979), *The Revolutions of Wisdom: Studies in the Claims and Practice of Ancient Greek Science* (1987) and *Demystifying Mentalities* (1990) all deal in detail with the language of proto-scientific writing and contain analysis of Hippocratic treatises as part of a wider project that explores the development of science more generally. Yet, these studies tend to separate argument from persuasion and overemphasise the importance of logical argument in early works of natural philosophy. In doing so, they miss some of the logic of mythic modes of expression which Detienne highlights.

Magic, Reason and Experience, for example, focuses on the interactions between traditional and more innovative, proto-scientific patterns of thought from the sixth to the fourth centuries BCE as a way of analysing the nature of the development of early Greek science. The first and second chapters of the book – 'The Criticism of Magic and the Inquiry Concerning Nature' and 'Dialectic and Demonstration' – examine the overlap and tensions between Pre-Socratic, medical and magico-religious modes of thought and then offer a detailed summary and exploration of the way that reasoning develops in philosophical, medical and mathematical writing, along with a discussion of the importance of persuasion.

In the first chapter, Lloyd explores connections between Pre-Socratic philosophers' criticisms of traditional religious beliefs and customs and the attacks against the same in *On the Sacred Disease* and other Hippocratic treatises. He argues that the understanding of nature that we find in the Hippocratic treatises and other fifth-century writing was radically different from how nature was understood in traditional religion. However, referring to the Hippocratic writers specifically, he rejects the idea that their pre-eminence was supported by a firmer empirical basis or by better cures for disease than their magico-religious counterparts. He claims that the Hippocratic authors could '– negatively – . . . undermine their opponents' doctrines by arguing that appeals to the gods were arbitrary and superfluous, and that secondary elaborations were indeed just that, excuses or screens for failure, and – positively – . . . offer an alternative explanatory framework' (Lloyd 1979: 57). Lloyd describes the positive accounts of disease causation in some Hippocratic treatises as products of the imagination:

> the element of over-optimism – or pure bluff – in the Hippocratics' own position is clear: many of their treatments were ineffectual and many of the correlations and causal connections they announced as fact (such as restriction of epilepsy to those of phlegmatic constitution) were imaginary.
> (Lloyd 1979: 57; see also Lloyd 1987: 15 for a similar statement)

Questions arise, however, about the nature of this 'bluff', this imaginative aspect to their work. How and why exactly did the Hippocratic authors seek to be convincing if, as Lloyd claims, they were covering up for ineffectual treatments and causal connections which are not supported by rational explanation or empirical evidence? Did the authors, as implied here, use reasoning in a way that was poorly prosecuted? Or is there something more going on in the positive account of the disease that we cannot easily appreciate if we label these accounts as 'poorly prosecuted'? Can we be sure, in other words, that the author has a model of 'well prosecuted reasoning' available in the first place? Indeed, since the author's explanatory framework is based neither on empirical data nor on better cures for disease, as Lloyd maintains, it is worthwhile trying to investigate the assumptions that underlie explanation in the treatise.

Lloyd makes the point that 'There is, as yet . . . no formal analysis of different modes of argument as such, no attempt expressly to define the distinction between necessary and probable reasoning, or that between proof and persuasion' (Lloyd 1979: 78). If this is the case, and for the Pre-Socratic, Sophistic and Hippocratic authors there is no clear notion of logical argument as opposed to 'mere' persuasion, how does it help us to understand their work better if we judge it as lacking in this respect?

One positive way to consider this issue further would be to examine early uses of words relating to argument, demonstration and proof. In *Demystifying Mentalities* Lloyd notes that a variety of nouns and verbs are used to refer to 'proving' in legal and other speculative contexts (he mentions, for example, the terms ἐπίδειξις, ἀποδείξις and δείκνυμι). He refers to *On the Nature of Human Beings*, quoting an extract from near the beginning of this work:

> In Ch. 2 (p. 170, line 3ff) the writer states: 'I for my part shall show [apodeixō] that the substances that I believe compose the human body are [. . .] always the same and unchanging: in youth and in old age, in cold weather as in warm. I shall produce proofs [anagkas] through which each thing is increased and decreased in the body.'
>
> (1990: 78)

Lloyd goes on to note that

> while the Hippocratic writer produces some good arguments to refute a rival view, when it comes to clinching the case for his own theory he is . . . much weaker. The main evidence he cites for his own element theory is that the four humours are all found in the excreta.
> (Ch. 5ff., p. 176 line 10ff., p. 180 line 2ff., p. 182 line 12ff) (1990: 79)

Here we have indications of the way in which a Hippocratic author seems to be engaging in logical argument; yet, if the arguments he uses to support his own theories are weak, why does he advertise them as 'proofs'? Is it that his argument, though weak, is still better than any of the others available at the time? Or could it be that the meanings of the terms ἀποδείξω 'I will demonstrate' and ἀνάγκας 'proofs' are still in the process of being thought through in this period? Would the listener or reader of this treatise have acknowledged the weakness of the ἀνάγκας 'proofs', or would this not have been the point, so much as the fact that the author states persuasively that he has ἀνάγκας 'proofs' and goes on to indicate them? The history of the use of these terms demands further clarification.

The relationship between style and thought in early Greek writing

A further area of scholarship which feeds into this discussion of the different modes of persuasion linked to argumentation is that of studies on style, such as Denniston (1960 [1952]), Dover (1997), Lilja (1968) and Wenskus (1982). As with the work of Hankinson and Lloyd above, these studies are influenced to a greater or lesser degree by what Thomas Cole describes in *The Origins of Rhetoric in Ancient Greece* as the notion of 'the absolute separability of a speaker's message from the method used to transmit it' (1991: 13), an essentially Platonic and Aristotelian invention and understanding of 'rhetoric'. In other words, the idea here is that meaning can be extricated from the form in which it is communicated, and by implication that form is subservient to meaning.

Denniston's study, published posthumously in incomplete form, usefully describes and categorises a range of common features of Greek prose writing, including abstract expression, word order, sentence structure, repetition, asyndeton and assonance; while these observations are helpful in building up a better understanding of the history of Greek prose style, there are relatively few attempts to analyse the persuasive function or effect of these features and so to grapple with the issue of their relationship with the development of Greek thought. Yet, Denniston tends to project moral judgements onto the authors considered, with criticism reserved for Gorgias; Gorgias nevertheless features as a landmark in the history of Greek prose writing. While the extensive discussion on features of form in this study tends to focus on the influence on the stylistic qualities of individual authors and of one author's style upon another's, discussion of persuasive function tends to be left aside, because of an underlying set of assumptions about what constitutes the best kind of prose.

For example, Denniston notes of Thucydides that 'The common craze for verbal antithesis is in him transformed into a craze for logical antithesis', arguing that in such cases 'the form controls the content, not the content the form' (1960 [1952]: 13). Gorgias, because of his emphasis on form, arguably over content (as if form and content could be neatly separated), is said to exaggerate balance and antithesis 'to the point of absurdity' and to have had a 'wholly bad' influence on Greek prose (1960 [1952]: 10). He continues: 'we are left wondering how it was that Gorgias, performing in the πρυτανεῖον τῆς σοφίας, before an audience whose taste had been educated by a century of great literature, was able to "get away with it"' (1960 [1952]: 12). The point here seems to be more that this idealising narrative of the development of Greek prose is inadequate to fully grapple with questions of aesthetic appreciation among the ancient Greeks. If, as Denniston implies, Gorgias was a linguistic radical in this era, then exactly what role did his radicalism play in the broader processes by which prose expression changed? Furthermore, how does this intersect with the intellectual revolutions taking place on a wider scale than the changes in linguistic style during this period?

Denniston does, nevertheless, acknowledge, along the lines of Detienne above, the mystical power of the word in earliest Greece:

> The prose of the early philosophers sets out to devise an elaborate word-music comparable to poetry in aesthetic value. It freely employs

alliteration and compound words which are not only impressive in their own nature but lend themselves to the production of assonance. Greater effect is given to these devices by the order of words, which is diversified and frequently chiastic. As prose technique develops, alliteration is felt to be crude, and passes out of fashion: while the separation of the language of poetry from that of prose limits a prose-writer's, or at any rate and orator's, freedom to use elaborate compounds as a basis of assonance. Simultaneously, the evolution of the highly polished Isocratean period, with symmetrically balanced clauses, encourages the growth of homoeoteleuton, which to a large extent ousts rival forms of assonance from the field, and replaces them by a system of rhymes so mechanical and monotonous as to make portions of Greek prose literature almost unreadable. In Plato, however, much of the old feeling for the mystical significance of words survives, and is to be detected particularly in the works of his old age; where it exists side by side with a delight, rather naïve from a modern point of view, in sound-echoes for their own sake.

(1960 [1952]: 139)

There are several value-judgements in this quotation, such as on the monotony of homoeoteleuton, which are problematic for any study into the function of persuasive features since the underlying question here – which it may not be possible to answer – is what effect did such features have on the ancient audiences, rather than on the modern reader's ear? Yet, the outline of the development of prose and incorporation of assonance as a signal to the mysticism of the word is an important point to consider when reading Hippocratic texts.

In *The Evolution of Greek Prose Style* (1997), Dover develops Denniston's work on style, working under the principal question 'how did Greek prose, with a long history of poetry behind it, evolve during the fifth and fourth centuries until – to borrow the expression used by Aristotle of mid-fifth-century tragedy – it 'attained its proper nature' in Plato and Demosthenes?' (1997: vi). In the study, Dover acknowledges different levels of style, explaining that while his study focuses on 'linguistic style' (1997: 11) there also exists 'style at the level of invention' (1997: 3), which is characterised by style being closely linked to thought processes and to action. There exists, however, a strong idealising and moralising streak in this book which can interfere with open analysis of the evidence: Platonic and Demosthenic constructions of 'proper' or 'best' in terms of prose writing referred to in the book's opening questions, cited above, are conflated with Dover's own aesthetic judgements. This is problematic because it implies insufficient critical distance from Plato's and Demosthenes' aesthetic and moral projects, not to mention their self-promotional activities, which in turn may skew our understanding of the development of early Greek prose writing.

This issue here is acknowledged to an extent, by Dover:

> We can agree that literature is an art-form, only to be beset by the even more forbidding question – also impossible to translate satisfactorily into Greek – 'What is art?' This question, however, becomes much less forbidding once we have succeeded in shaking free of the common notion that art is always and necessarily good, a notion that leads to the dismissal of some literature, painting, and music as 'not art'. It is preferable to begin with the acknowledgement that a very great number of works of art are trivial, incompetent, worthless, of such a kind that our emotional response to them is much less favourable than our response to natural phenomena or even to patterns and sequences of sounds and sights which result from an accident. After that we can start to think about what makes good art.
>
> (1997: 22)

However, it is not necessary, and seems to me unhelpful, to form judgements about the quality of any product of expression in order to make critical enquiries about its expressive intention.

Dover's study also contains many essential insights into and a deep knowledge of examples of early prose writing. On the issue of the distinction between form and content, Dover helpfully notes: 'Dogmatic answers have sometimes been given to the unhelpful question "Can form and content be separated?", when the question which matters is "To what extent, and in what circumstances, is it useful to separate form from content?"' (1997: 12). The question is pertinent to this study, to which an attempted answer is given for the purposes of dealing with Hippocratic texts in the form of the analysis of the five Hippocratic treatises in the following chapters.

There are also insights on the range of prose models available to early authors, on units of sense, on rhythm, structure, vocabulary, genre and linguistic dialect and geographical locations in which early prose developed which are in different ways pertinent to this discussion and will be referred to as appropriate in what follows. The study aims generally at statistical data which can help to form a more thoroughgoing empirical account of the evolution of Greek prose, rather than to ask questions about the persuasive function and effects of such work, though again there are occasional comments which are directly relevant to this discussion.

In terms of methodological support for this study, Dover's discussion of the point that no piece of writing can have no style and that there is no *a priori* limit to the number of ways two texts can be compared stylistically is important here (1997: 43). Dover notes that because of the absence of any preconceived criterion by which texts can be judged stylistically, 'we shall be wise to begin from those which strike us as unusual and to discover whether our impression is correct' (1997: 43); such is the method employed in this analysis.

Rosalind Thomas' work on Herodotus' *Histories* and its intellectual milieu, which does achieve an analysis incorporating attention to form as well as content, aims to reserve judgement about the aesthetic value or effectiveness of such writing and considers the presence of different levels of 'logic' or argumentation being employed within the same work. Thomas examines how Herodotus' use of the language of argument in Book II should be understood as part of the late fifth-century BCE world of developing use of argumentation. Herodotus is engaging in this book in contemporary debates about nature that relate back to Pre-Socratic thinkers and which continue beyond him, and are also used by the Hippocratic authors in their medical treatises (Thomas 2000: 60–75).

In Chapter 6 of *Herodotus in Context,* entitled 'Argument and the Language of Proof', Thomas examines Herodotus' analytical mode, noting that little work has been carried out on this topic and that earlier work is sometimes problematic because it focuses on the truth value of the arguments that Hero-dotus is making, rather than the methods he employs in arguing. (Thomas 2000: 172–173).

Through exploring several examples of the use of claims to proof in the *Histories*, she argues that the uses move in the direction of persuasion and away from testable demonstrations supported by evidence:

> This is a style which flaunted the presence of evidence and proofs for the theory in question, and which begins to have an overtly rhetorical edge: such claims have become the necessary claims to make, whatever the nature of your evidence.
>
> (Thomas 2000: 198)

For Thomas,

> argument of the type known as *modus tollens*, that is: If A, then B; but not B; therefore not A – a type of deductive argument not formally expressed in general terms until Aristotle but used well before; the enthymeme; argument from likelihood (*eikos*); listing of arguments; explicit citation of evidence or 'proof' as part of this; *reductio ad absurdum*; argument from analogy; *a fortiori* reasoning
>
> (2000: 175)

are all part of the *persuasive* resources of Herodotus in grappling with questions about the nature of the river Nile.

The inclusion of these features associated with scientific method does not necessarily denote adherence to a scientific method; rather, Thomas argues, they indicate a style of approach to questions of natural philosophy and a flamboyant display of allegiance to contemporary trends: 'for Herodotus, the claim to have 'proofs' often signals some of his most complex or most controversial ideas'; '*Tekmeria* certainly do not involve empirical evidence, if by 'empirical' one means evidence from experience, or from sight, or evidence that can be tested, though they do involve evidence of some kind' (Thomas 2000: 193).

Thomas also notes the accompaniment of the use of these argument terms with features associated with persuasion in poetry, as, for example, with Parmenides' invocation of a poetic goddess in his poem on truth and with Empedocles' invocation of the muse in his poem on nature (2000: 198 f.).

Thomas' analysis of Herodotus' use of argumentation is highly convincing and includes attention to logical inference as well as more subjective persuasive elements. There is also discussion in the study of a similar phenomenon in Hippocratic treatises, which Thomas argues are part of the same late fifth-century world of public debate on issues of natural philosophy (e.g. Thomas 2000: 178–182; 185–189). Yet there are also further persuasive aspects to Herodotus' and his contemporaries' writing that are not evident from an analysis of persuasive use of argumentative techniques alone, attention to which can help us to better understand the nature of this phase in the development of prose.

There is not only an overlap in terms of 'mere' persuasion in the use of argument terms, but a more positive persuasive element, involving patterning features present in early Greek prose writing, than Thomas allows for in her study. By letting go of the association between argument and logical argumentation in reading display prose of this period, we open up to a world in which references to proofs and evidence are only some among a rich treasury of persuasive features which sought to convince and, for all we know, may well have convinced ancient audiences and which may all have a kind of logic underpinning them. We can attempt therefore to uncover the personal logic(s) that are expressed in individual enquiries into nature, enquiries which embrace both the poetic and the (pseudo-)scientific.

Models of explanation in early Greek writing

In the above we have seen, then, that while *On the Sacred Disease* represents a major advance in scientific thinking because of the way that it includes examples of logical thinking which are considered philosophically robust, it also shows signs of making use of other modes of logic or patterning to convince its intended audience, which may derive from mythic narratives.

We have also seen how it is problematic for form – or style – to be separated from content in discussions of early Greek prose writing, for in many ways this goes against the grain of the expressive aims and interests of fifth-century authors.

In order to tune into the Hippocratic notion of explanation we need to become adept at paying attention to their methods of persuasion, temporarily leaving aside more modern notions of explanation and of validity.[7] A reassessment of the persuasive aims of Hippocratic oratory in light of models of argumentative persuasion in the period is required if we are to gain insight into the spirit of the period in which they were composed.

In the following section of this chapter, building on the examples for models of Hippocratic oratory cited briefly in the first chapter, I will outline examples of some of the most influential and prominent models of persuasive argument in the late fifth century BCE and shortly before, and identify some of the ways that poetics – the formal features and style of writing – have a hand in the process of arguing a case or a point of view.

(a) Parmenides' 'Way of truth'

One significant early example of description of a path towards truth, which must have been an influence on the development of explanations in expository prose, is found in Parmenides' work. Here we find a description of a journey towards truth conveyed through metaphor and in verse form that foreshadows the notion of necessary consequence that is key to the Aristotelian definition of argument in *Prior Analytics* and thus gives us a hint as to how ideas about valid and invalid explanation were developing in the period prior to Aristotle. As noted earlier in this chapter, Detienne explores this poem from the point of view of its use of earlier pre-rational structures of meaning. Here, I focus solely on how the poem anticipates the language of logical explanation in prose which develops in later decades in ancient Greece.

The following extract is taken from the extant prologue to Parmenides' poem, which is today considered to have consisted of two parts, the 'Way of Truth' and the 'Way of Appearance'. In this prologue, Parmenides describes a journey on a carriage led by the daughters of the sun from the world of daylight into a world of night where a goddess addresses him as follows:

ὦ κοῦρ᾽ ἀθανάτῃσι συνήορος ἡνιόχοισιν,
ἵπποις θ᾽ αἵ σε φέρουσιν ἱκάνων ἡμέτερον δῶ,
χαῖρ᾽, ἐπεὶ οὔτι σε μοῖρα κακὴ προύπεμπε νέεσθαι
τήνδ᾽ ὁδόν, ἦ γὰρ ἀπ᾽ ἀνθρώπων ἐκτὸς πάτου ἐστίν,
ἀλλὰ Θέμις τε Δίκη τε. χρεὼ δέ σε πάντα πυθέσθαι
ἠμὲν Ἀληθείης εὐκυκλέος ἀτρεμὲς ἦτορ
ἠδὲ βροτῶν δόξας . . .

O youth, companion to immortal charioteers,
and to mares which bear you, as you arrive at our abode,
hail! since no evil fate sent you forth to travel
this way (for indeed it is far from the track of men),
but Right and Justice. It is right for you to learn all things,
both the unshaken heart of well-rounded Truth,
and the opinions of mortals . . .

(TEGP 210–213 (10 F1) = DK28B1, 24–32 [adapted])[8]

There is an extensive discussion that could be entered into about this passage that cannot be considered here. However, from the point of view of the development of argumentation in explanation, it is the first explicit expression that we have in our sources of the idea that a journey along a certain path through abstract concepts can lead to another place where there is a greater level of insight available. The journey is one which is described as presided over by 'Right and Justice' and is led by the daughters of the sun, so it is a well-defined path; indeed, defined by forces beyond the control of the young man in question. The speaker implies that the young man has arrived by means of his companionship with the immortal charioteers and mares that have transported him. This could be read as a metaphor for the way argument leads one to certain conclusions and as such operates independently of the user of argument to some extent. The journey, we are told, was prompted by 'Right and Justice', which are personifications of abstract notions. We could understand the prompting of these divine figures in secular terms as a desire to know the truth.

'Truth' is characterised in the extract as 'εὐκυκλέος' 'well-rounded'.[9] This is important because it emphasises the form which 'truth' is thought to take and suggests a preconception about what truth looks like and its connection with symmetry and unity. Similarly, the description 'ἀτρεμὲς ἦτορ' 'steady heart' suggests fixity and vital importance: these descriptions bring us towards the idea of a notion of truth defined by aesthetic qualities.

This sense of truth as having a particular form is further explained in other fragments of Parmenides' work, which make reference to a particular path to truth being pursued by reasoning, with signs indicating the way to truth, and give more substance to Parmenides' understanding of the notion of 'truth' as 'what-is'. For example:

κρῖναι δὲ λόγωι πολύδηριν ἔλεγχον
ἐξ ἐμέθεν ῥηθέντα

But judge by reasoning the very contentious examination
uttered by me.

(TEGP 214–215 (16 [F7]) = DK28B7, 5–6)[10]

and

> μόνος δ᾽ἔτι μῦθος ὁδοῖο
> λείπεται ὡς ἔστιν· ταύτηι δ᾽ἐπὶ σήματ᾽ἔασι
> πολλὰ μάλ᾽, ὡς ἀγένητον ἐὸν καὶ ἀνώλεθρόν ἐστιν,
> οὖλον μουνογενές τε καὶ ἀτρεμὲς ἠδὲ τέλειον.

> Only one tale is left of the way:
> that it is; and on this are posted
> very many signs, that what-is is ungenerated and imperishable,
> a whole of one kind, unperturbed and complete.
> (TEGP 214–217 (17 [F8]) = DK28B8, 1–4)[11]

There are many elements of this extract from Parmenides' proem (i.e. the opening, introductory section of his poem) that do not obviously relate to later Hippocratic material. The use of divine figures in the description of the journey towards 'truth' is not something we find in other early expository contexts. However, Parmenides' work does highlight certain themes – the notion of a *journey* towards 'truth' and the sense of 'truth' having a particular form – that we will see picked up in the discussion of features of expression in the following chapters. The descriptions 'well-rounded' and 'complete' could perhaps be replaced with 'watertight', an adjective that is used today in describing a sound argument and which has a special resonance for the persuasive work of all the early authors.[12]

(b) Heraclitus' experiments with form

In terms of experimentation with language, and with the play on the shift from prose to poetry, a key early author whose influence persists in much Sophistic and some Hippocratic work is the Pre-Socratic philosopher Heraclitus, writing near the beginning of the fifth century BCE in the eastern Aegean. Though Heraclitus' philosophical approach to the notion of *logos* is at odds with Parmenides' – as discussed in much detail in scholarship on the topic – it is important to include him in this introduction to styles of writing, for Heraclitus sets a tone for the kinds of wilder experiments with meaning through play on language that characterise certain 'oral' Hippocratic treatises, much Sophistic writing and sections of the work of Herodotus.[13]

In the maxims cited below, Heraclitus offers a subtle vision of nature that involves, among other ideas, a notion of unity in opposition which is conveyed through intricate fusion of form and content. Heraclitus remarks: 'ποταμοῖσι τοῖσιν αὐτοῖσιν ἐμβαίνουσιν ἕτερα καὶ ἕτερα ὕδατα ἐπιρρεῖ' 'On those stepping into the same rivers other and other waters flow' (TEGP 158–159

(62 [F39]) = DK22B12) and that the river 'σκίδνησι καὶ πάλιν συνάγει . . . συνίσταται καὶ ἀπολείπει καὶ πρόσεισι καὶ ἄπεισι' 'scatters things and in turn regathers them . . . it comes together and separates . . . approaches and departs' (TEGP 158–159 (66) = DK22B91)[14] He plays here with the idea of change and permanence, highlighting the fact that the river is at once 'the same river' and yet that it continually changes through clever phrasing that reflects and enhances the overall meaning of his statements. The word 'ἕτερα' means 'different [waters]' and so indicates change, but its repetition in the sentence signals permanence. Similarly, the three oppositions 'scatters and regathers, comes together and separates, approaches and departs' here describe change, but in their form show similarity in that they are all oppositions. Heraclitus, then, set a standard for the manipulation of form to communicate meaning whose influence can arguably be detected in the most elaborate examples of subsequent expository prose writing.[15]

Heraclitus' intense focus on form reminds us of the point that expository prose is born out of expository verse writing. For an insight into the first major example of extended prose in the ancient Greek world, we must turn to Herodotus, the second book of whose *Histories* contains debates on the nature of the Nile that are widely recognised now as showing a close connection with Pre-Socratic and Hippocratic debates about natural phenomena.[16]

(c) Herodotus' enquiries into the nature of the Nile

Herodotus' work covers expanses of time, space and, from a modern point of view, genre. His overall theme is the causes of the Greco-Persian conflict and he tells us that he is writing 'ὡς μήτε τὰ γενόμενα ἐξ ἀνθρώπων τῷ χρόνῳ ἐξίτηλα γένηται, μήτε ἔργα μεγάλα τε καὶ θωμαστά, τὰ μὲν Ἕλλησι τὰ δὲ βαρβάροισι ἀποδεχθέντα, ἀκλεᾶ γένηται' 'in order that the memory of the past may not be blotted out from among people by time and that great and marvellous deeds done by Greeks and foreigners may not lack renown' (*Histories* I, 1) As part of his *Histories*, Herodotus devotes the second of his nine books to a discussion of the earliest known history of Egypt, the nature of the country and the customs of its people.[17] Here, among Herodotus' enquiries about the first kings of Egypt and the antiquity of the Egyptian language, we find a discussion of the geographical feature of Egypt which is most important from the point of view of human settlement there: the river Nile. This discussion resembles the writing of earlier natural philosophers in many ways – indeed, Herodotus is contributing to ongoing debate about the river Nile since we know that some Pre-Socratic thinkers also wrote about the nature of the Nile.[18]

One example of his discussion at this point in the *Histories* is his argument for the claim that Egypt once did not exist and the deposits of the Nile created its land. In the following extract from this discussion we can see echoes of earlier authors and at the same time a distinct method of argumentation:

Ἔστι δὲ τῆς Ἀραβίης χώρης, Αἰγύπτού δὲ οὐ πρόσω, κόλπος θαλάσσης ἐσέχων ἐκ τῆς Ἐρυθρῆς καλεομένης θαλάσσης, μακρὸς οὕτω δή τι καὶ στεινὸς ὡς ἔρχομαι φράσων· μῆκος μὲν πλόου ἀρξαμένῳ ἐκ μυχοῦ διεκπλῶσαι ἐς τὴν εὐρέαν θάλασσαν ἡμέραι ἀναισιμοῦνται τεσσεράκοντα εἰσεσίη χρεωμένῳ· εὖρος δέ, τῇ εὐρύτατος ἐστὶ ὁ κόλπος, ἥμισυ ἡμέρης πλόου. ῥηχίη δ᾽ ἐν αὐτῷ καὶ ἄμπωτις ἀνὰ πᾶσαν ἡμέρην γίνεται. ἕτερον τοιοῦτον κόλπον καὶ τὴν Αἴγυπτον δοκέω γενέσθαι κοτέ, τὸν μὲν ἐκ τῆς βορηίης θαλάσσης κόλπον ἐσέχοντα επ᾽ Αἰθιοπίης, τὸν δὲ Ἀράβιον, τὸν ἔρχομαι λέξων, ἐκ τῆς νοτίης φέροντα ἐπὶ Συρίης, σχεδὸν μὲν ἀλλήλοισι συντετραίνοντας τοὺς μυχούς, ὀλίγον δέ τι παραλλάσσοντας τῆς χώρης.

Now in Arabia, not far from Egypt, there is a gulf of the sea entering in from the sea called Red, of which the length and narrowness is such as I shall show: for length, it is a forty days' voyage for a ship rowed by oars from its inner end out to the wide sea; and for breadth, it is half a day's voyage at the widest. Every day the tide ebbs and flows therein. I hold that where now is Egypt there was once another such gulf; one entered from the northern sea towards Aethiopia, and the other, the Arabian gulf of which I will speak, bore from the south towards Syria; the ends of these gulfs pierced into the country near to each other, and but a little space of land divided them.[19]

(*Histories*, II, 11)

Here we can see Herodotus arguing for the idea that the geographical area he considers Egypt was once a gulf of the sea by analogy with the gulf of the Red Sea. He suggests that the course of the Nile traces the central line of a large gulf that once existed, narrowing southwards from where Egypt today meets the Mediterranean Sea at the Nile Delta. Herodotus highlights the point that these gulfs are imagined as being geographically opposite in direction: Herodotus describes one as cutting in from the Mediterranean Sea towards Aethiopia and the other from the south towards Syria.

There is symmetry of shape, direction and extent to the two gulfs that Herodotus is describing here. There are other features of this description that work towards creating patterns. Notice how Herodotus picks up on the action of the seawater in describing the Red Sea: 'ῥηχίη δ᾽ ἐν αὐτῷ καὶ ἄμπωτις ἀνὰ πᾶσαν ἡμέρην γίνεται' 'Every day the tide ebbs and flows therein'. This is a way of anticipating through a suggestive hint the conclusion that he is about to draw: the continually changing movement of the sea is conjured up in an image to prepare us for the notion that a great change has taken place to the country of Egypt as a result of the movement of water. This attention to the power of water also anticipates Herodotus' discussion, later on in the same book, of the flooding of the Nile.

In describing the two gulfs, Herodotus states that 'σχεδὸν μὲν ἀλλήλοισι συντετραίνοντας τοὺς μύχούς, ὀλίγον δέ τι παραλλάσσοντας τῆς χώρης' 'the ends of these gulfs pierced into the country near to each other, and but a little space of land divided them'. The gulfs are almost touching one another, the word 'ἀλλήλοισι' 'to each other' implying that there is a connection between these two gulfs and therefore reinforcing through seemly explanation the notion that both of these two gulfs existed, recalling the symmetry of their shape, direction and extent. The pervasive idea underlying this description is that the natural world can be understood through patterns – analogies and symmetries.[20]

In this example from the *Histories*, from the point of view of argument in explanation, this concentration of patterning connects with Parmenides' description, or rather personification, of truth's heart as 'εὐκυκλέος' 'well-rounded' and as 'ἀτρεμές' 'steady'. The sense of there being one single valid explanation also comes across in Herodotus' theory about the action of the river Nile: Herodotus does not admit additional factors to his theory. The truth has a certain shape, therefore, in Herodotus' account; however, unlike in Parmenides' account of the process of reasoning, in Herodotus' account the force of his argument comes as much from associative connections and suggestions as from strict logic.

The examples cited above seem to confirm the sense that while notions of valid explanation are being developed in the fifth century BCE, there is a high degree of exploration and experimentation involved in this process and that there is no one agreed standard for valid argument.

(d) On Breaths

Let us finally turn to some features of expression connected with the notion of explanation and argument from *On Breaths* that will be the subject of further examination in subsequent chapters.

In the following passage from the middle of the treatise, the author is discussing the second of the two types of fever he claims exist in the world: 'individual' fever, which affects those individuals who follow a bad regimen. The author is assuming as a general unargued proposition that internal crises can be caused by the entry of elements/items from outside, asserting that shivering is a case in point. At this point in the discussion, which leads up to a description of the development of shivering, the author notes the kinds of regimen that can bring about internal crises and also comments how excess air, which is key to the development of shivering, enters the body.

τοῦτο μὲν ὅταν τις πλέονας τροφάς, ὑγρὰς ἢ ξηράς, διδοῖ τῷ σώματι ἢ τὸ σῶμα δύναται φέρειν καὶ πόνον μηδένα τῷ πλήθει τῶν τροφέων ἀντιτιθῇ, τοῦτο δ᾽ὅταν ποικίλας καὶ ἀνομοίους ἀλλήλησιν ἐσπέμπη τροφάς· τὰ γὰρ ἀνόμοια στασιάζει, καὶ τὰ μὲν θᾶσσον, τὰ δὲ σχολαίτερον πέσσεται. Μετὰ δὲ πολλῶν σιτίων ἀνάγκη καὶ πολλὸν πνεῦμα ἐσιέναι.

this [happens] on the one hand whenever more food, moist or dry, is given to the body than the body can bear, without counteracting the bulky food by exercise; on the other hand whenever foods that are varied and dissimilar are taken. For dissimilar foods disagree, and some are digested quickly and some more slowly. Now along with much food much wind too must enter.

(On Breaths, 7.1–2)

The causal link between bad regimen and internal crisis is expressed here through the ordering of description, the use and mutual reinforcement of key terms such as 'ἀνόμοιος' 'dissimilar', 'ποικίλος' 'various' 'ἀλλήλων' 'of one another' while citing an external piece of evidence (i.e., that dissimilar foods disagree). We can also note an accumulation of words for quantity which all – perhaps coincidentally – sound similar: 'πλέονας' 'πλήθει' 'πολλῶν' 'πολλὸν'. The author also employs the well-known and charged political term 'στασιάζω' 'to form a party or faction' to describe internal crises, emphasising the point further that the language being used here is working to project a vision of workings of physiology on to the body which seems likely to have its evidential basis, insofar as it has one, in lived political experiences.

Another extract from *On Breaths* again shows persuasive language at work in supporting a claim. In the following extract, the author is discussing the role of 'flux' or 'discharge' 'τὰ ῥεύματα' (which seems to mean a downward flowing of certain fluid(s) – usually 'τὸ φλέγμα' through the body) as agents of disease and defending the claim that air is also the primary cause of discharge. Here, the author is describing what happens once air trapped in the head has triggered a discharge:

Ὅπῃ δ᾽ ἂν ἀθρόον ἀφίκηται τοῦ σώματος, ἐνταῦθα σύνίσταται ἡ νοῦσος. Ἢν μὲν οὖν ἐπὶ τὴν ὄψιν ἔλθῃ, ταύτῃ ὁ πόνος· ἢν δὲ ἐς τὰς ἀκοάς, ἐνταῦθα ἡ νοῦσος· ἢν δ᾽ ἐς τὰς ῥῖνας, κόρυζα· ἢν δ᾽ ἐς τὰ στέρνα, βράγχος καλεῖται· τὸ γὰρ φλέγμα δριμέσιν χυμοῖσιν μεμιγμένον, ὅπῃ ἂν προσπέσῃ ἐς ἀήθεας τόπους, ἑλκοῖ·

Any part of the body that it reaches in mass becomes the seat of a disease. If it goes to the eyes, the pain is there; if it be to the ears, the disease is there. If it goes to the nose, coryza occurs. If it goes to the chest, it is called sore throat; for phlegm, mixed with acrid humours, produces sores wherever it strikes an unusual spot.

(*On Breaths*, 10, 2)[21]

The rapid listing of possible places the mass of 'phlegm' can afflict highlights the sense of invasion of the inner space of the body. The listing device also sends out the impression that the author is noting a wide range of possible eventualities in his description; just as the 'phlegm' itself is powerful because it is the agent of a variety of ailments, so the explanation, because it focuses on the 'phlegm', has the power to explain the occurrence of all these ailments. The final line of this extract, suggesting that other ailments are simply permutations of the same basic agent – phlegm mixed with acrid humours produces sores – further helps to suggest that the author holds the expository key to all illnesses.

Both of these extracts from *On Breaths* can be linked back to the notion of argument leading to truth that we saw depicted in the extract from Parmenides and to Herodotus' emphasis on patterning in explanation. Here, as before, persuasive features of language build up patterns and structures which are employed to support the claims being made in each case and elaborate upon initial propositions.

We are looking in these examples of early prose, at a certain *way* of discussing theories of nature, of expressing the notion of journey towards the truth and of supporting argument that is common to these authors. It is this sense of a kinship in mode of expression, as well as the underlying sense of persuasive efficacy and of understanding of nature that this implies, that also characterises Hippocratic oratory.

We have seen, then, in this chapter, how it is limiting to read strictly defined notions of argument in the philosophical tradition following on from Aristotle's work into Hippocratic treatises because doing so causes other layers of meaning and manners of conveying truth claims to be obscured. Furthermore, we have seen how analysis of Greek prose that assumes a clean distinction between style and content and avoids examining the relationship between form and a work's overall meaning limits and skews our understanding of the expressive endeavours of early Greek prose writing, including Hippocratic writing.

We have also seen how looser notions of logic or logics through which meaning is conveyed by patterns of association, which may be expressed in written or other form and which derive from earlier mythic modes of meaning, are an important model for Hippocratic prose writing. It has become clear, through an analysis of examples of Parmenides', Heraclitus' and Herodotus' work that key Hippocratic texts are building on from their predecessors' work and mix truth claims with expressive patterning in order to build a case. Such writing cannot be fully appreciated if read reductively for its expression of ideas that obey rational principles.

In the next chapter, I explore further the evidence for the nature of Hippocratic expository prose and for its delivery context and persuasive function. I consider how far the genre of *epideixis* is relevant in studying Hippocratic oratorical texts and consider evidence for the orality of Hippocratic oratory, that is persuasive features which suggest an affinity with the tradition of oral dissemination of ideas.

Notes

1 See, for example, Stesichorus on the standard version of the story of Helen: 'οὐκ ἔστ᾽ἔτυμος λόγος οὗτος, / οὐδ᾽ἔβας ἐν νηυσὶν ἐϋςςέλμοις / οὐδ᾽ ἵκεο πέργαμα Τροίας.' 'That story is not true: / you did not go on the well-benched ships / and you did not reach the citadel of Troy' fr. 192 (Davies 1991: 177–179); Pindar on the standard version of the story of the eating of Pelops in *Olympian* I: 'ἦ θαύματα πολλά, καί πού τι καὶ βροτῶν / φάτις ὑπὲρ τὸν ἀλαθῆ λόγον / δεδαιδαλμένοι ψεύδεσι ποικίλοις / ἐξαπατῶντι μῦθοι.' 'Yes, wonders are many, but then too, I think, in men's talk / stories are embellished beyond the true account / and deceive by means of / elaborate lies' (Race 1997: ll. 28a–29).

2 Another important example of recent discussion of *logos* in scholarship on ancient philosophy is Schofield and Nussbaum (1982).

3 'Aletheia and Lethe are not exclusive or contradictory ways of thinking; they constitute two extremes of a single religious power' (Detienne 1996: 16) and, also on the same pairing, 'The positive tends toward the negative, which, in a way, "denies" it but cannot maintain itself in its absence' (Detienne 1996: 82).

4 See also e.g. Longrigg (1993) and Powell (2007).

5 As analysed in detail in van der Eijk (2005).

6 In Laskaris (2002: 539–550).

7 Cole notes in the preface to his book, which gives an account of and analyses the development of persuasion towards the philosophical notions of rhetoric conveyed and discussed in the work of Plato and Aristotle: 'The rhetoric of my title and of the investigation that follows is rhetoric in the narrowest and most conventional sense of the term: a speaker's or writer's self-conscious manipulation of his medium with a view to ensuring his message as favorable a reception as possible on the part of the particular audience being addressed. The self-consciously manipulative character of the process distinguishes rhetoric from eloquence, which may be unpremeditated and stem from nothing more than a natural knack for clear and expressive utterance; orientation towards communicational goal distinguishes rhetoric from the type of verbal virtuosity in which the exploration or display of the resources of a given medium becomes an end in itself; indifference to the inherent character or value of the messages communicated so long as they are put across effectively distinguishes it from some of its modern namesakes – notably those which, in the wake of the twentieth-century 'revival' of the subject, would make of rhetoric either an overall science of discourse or an art of practical reasoning and deliberation.' (1991: ix) He views persuasive techniques, then, as part of the coming to consciousness of the science of rhetoric; see Chapters 7 'Rhetoric and Prose' and 8 'Rhetoric and Philosophy' of his book for analysis of the relationship between persuasive techniques and the development of dialectic and logical inference.

8 Cited in Sextus *Against the Professors*; lines 28–32 in Simplicius *On the Heavens*; and lines 28–30 in Diogenes Laertius. Note that TEGP quotes 'εὐπειθέος' 'persuasive' in place of 'εὐκυκλέος' 'well-rounded' found in Simplicius; 'εὐφεγγέος' 'bright-shining' is found in Proclus.

9 See note 8 above.

10 Cited in Sextus *Against the Professors* and Diogenes Laertius.

11 Cited in Simplicius *Physics* and lines 1–2 in Sextus *Against the Professors* etc.

12 Parmenides also emphatically uses the language of compulsion later on in his work as in DK28B7, for example: 'εἶργε' 'hold back' (line 2); 'βιάσθω' 'force' (line 3) and in DK28B8: 'οὐδ . . . ἐάσσω' 'I will not allow' (line 7), 'ἀπέσβεσται' 'is extinguished' (line 21), 'Ἀνάγκη' 'Necessity' (line 30) 'ἐν δεσμοῖσιν' 'in bonds' (line 31) which also communicate this sense of travelling along a fixed course.

13 See, for example, Verdenius (1966–1967). It is important to point out at this stage that one serious problem in dealing with the Pre-Socratic fragments as evidence for language use in early Greece is the distinction between the authentic words of the authors and secondary reports, which can be difficult to draw (see e.g. Runia 2008: 27–54). This is particularly the case with prose: in a chapter on the problem of the reliability of sources containing Pre-Socratic fragments, R. Sharples remarks that 'It is intrinsically more difficult in the case of references to an author writing in prose to distinguish between an actual report and its context, and to decide whether a report is verbatim quotation (except where this is explicitly indicated in the ancient source) than it is in the case of prose writers quoting from poetical authors' (2005: 432). Only those fragments considered authentic in the standard Diels-Kranz edition of the Pre-Socratics – labelled as 'B' fragments – are used as evidence in this book (Diels, 1964). While this does not overcome the issue of the authenticity of the texts cited, neither does it negate the significance of any parallels in language use observed between the Pre-Socratics and contemporary authors, though it does limit the certainty with which we can speak of influence of one author's language use upon another.

14 The first quotation (DK22B12) is cited in Eusebius *Preparation for the Gospel* and Arius Didymus; the second (DK22B91) is cited in Plutarch in *On the E at Delphi*.

15 Heraclitus' style was, however, considered problematic by later authors in search of clarity of thought and diction. Aristotle's *Rhetoric* 1407b11–18 (A4) notes: 'In general writing should be easy to read and to phrase. These are manifestations of the same quality – one which is lost when words make too many connections, and are difficult to punctuate, as in the writings of Heraclitus. For it is difficult to punctuate his text because it is unclear whether a word goes with what follows or what precedes. For instance, in the beginning of his treatise, he says 'Of this Word's being forever do men prove to be uncomprehending'. It is unclear which phrase 'forever' <should> go with.[Demetrius] *On Style* 191–192 notes: 'Clarity results from many words, first from referring terms, then from conjunctions. Text without conjunctions and completely unconnected is utterly unclear. For the beginning of each phrase is unclear owing to the lack of connection, as in Heraclitus' writing. For in fact the lack of connection makes it unclear for the most part' (Graham 2010: 141).

16 See, for example, Thomas (2000) as the most engaging and authoritative entry-point into this topic.

17 The literal translation of the noun 'ἱστορίη', which occurs in the first line of his work and is commonly used as the basis for the modern title '*Histories*' is 'a learning by inquiry'. The literal translation retains a better sense of the overall scope of Herodotus' work.

18 Herodotus mentions other contributors to the problem of the Nile flooding at 2, 20 f.; the different opinions have been attributed by scholars to Thales and Anaxagoras, but on precisely what grounds I have failed to see (see DK11A16 and DK59A91). On surer ground, Seneca *Natural Questions* 4a.2.22 (=DK22A11) notes that Thales grappled with the problem of explaining the flooding of the Nile. Anaxagoras is also said to have touched on this problem: see DK59A42. Democritus is also said to have engaged with the problem of why the Nile floods: see DK68A99.

19 It may also be that there are connections in terms of vocabulary between the medical writings and Herodotus here; 'συντετραίνω' 'to pierce [a channel]' in the passage above is also attested in *Airs, Waters, Places* 2.42, 3, for instance, so has a parallel in medical usage.

20 See Thomas (2006) for a discussion of the affinity of this section of Herodotus' *Histories* with contemporary prose, and specifically pseudo-scientific writing. See further Thomas (2000) on this topic.

21 'Coryza' refers to nasal congestion, a symptom of the common cold.

References

Cole, T. (1991), *The Origins of Rhetoric in Ancient Greece*. Baltimore, MD; London: The John Hopkins University Press.

Davies, M. (*ed. post* D. L. Page) (1991), *Poetarum Melicorum Graecorum Fragmenta*. Oxford, Oxford University Press.

Denniston, J. D. (1960 [1952]), *Greek Prose Style*. Oxford: Clarendon Press.

Detienne, M. (1996), *The Masters of Truth in Archaic Greece*; translated by J. Lloyd. New York: Zone Books; Cambridge, MA: Distributed by the MIT Press.

Diels, H. (1964), *Die Fragmente der Vorsokratiker: griechisch und deutsch.* Zurich; Berlin: Weidmann.

Dover, K. J. (1997), *The Evolution of Greek Prose Style*. Oxford: Clarendon Press.

van der Eijk, Ph. J. (2005), 'The "Theology" of the Hippocratic Treatise *On the Sacred Disease*' in van der Eijk, Ph. J. (ed.), *Medicine and Philosophy in Classical Antiquity. Doctors and Philosophers on Nature, Soul, Health and Disease*. Cambridge; New York: Cambridge University Press, 45–73 [first published in *Apeiron* 23 (1990), 87–119].

Graham, D. W. (2010), *The Texts of Early Greek Philosophy: The Complete Fragments and Selected Testimonies of the Major Presocratics*. Cambridge: Cambridge University Press.

Hankinson, R. J. (1998), *Cause and Explanation in Ancient Greek Thought*. Oxford: Clarendon Press.

Laskaris, J. (2002), *The Art Is Long: On the Sacred Disease and the Scientific Tradition*. Leiden; Boston, MA: Brill.

Lilja, S. (1968), *On the Style of the Earliest Greek Prose*. Helsinki: Societas Humanarum Fennica.

Lloyd, G. E. R. (1990), *Demystifying Mentalities*. Cambridge; New York: Cambridge University Press.

Lloyd, G. E. R. (1987), *The Revolutions of Wisdom: Studies in the Claims and Practice of Ancient Greek Science*. Berkeley: University of California Press.

Lloyd, G. E. R. (1979), *Magic, Reason, and Experience: Studies in the Origin and Development of Greek Science*. Cambridge: Cambridge University Press.

Lloyd, G. E. R. (1966), *Polarity and Analogy: Two Types of Argumentation in Early Greek Thought*. Cambridge: Cambridge University Press.

Longrigg, J. (1993), *Greek Rational Medicine: Philosophy and Medicine from Alcmaeon to the Alexandrians*. London; New York: Routledge.

Powell, J. (ed.) (2007), *Logos: Rational Argument in Classical Rhetoric*. London: University of London, School of Advanced Study, Institute of Classical Studies.

Purtill, R. (1995), 'Argument' in Audi, R. (ed.), *The Cambridge Dictionary of Philosophy*. Cambridge: Cambridge University Press. 37.

Race, W. H. (ed. and trans.) (1997), *Pindar: Olympian Odes, Pythian Odes*. Cambridge, MA; London, England: Harvard University Press.

Runia, D. T. (2008), 'The Sources for Pre-Socratic Philosophy' in Curd, P. and Graham, D. W. (eds.), *The Oxford Handbook of Pre-Socratic Philosophy*. Oxford: Oxford University Press. 27–54.

Schofield, M. and Nussbaum, M. (eds.) (1982), *Language and Logos: Studies in Ancient Greek Philosophy Presented to G. E. L. Owen*. Cambridge; New York: Cambridge University Press.

Sharples, R. W. (2005), 'The Problem of Sources' in Gil, M. L. and Pellegrin, P. (eds.), *A Companion to Ancient Philosophy*. Malden, MA; Oxford: Blackwell. 430–447.

Thomas, R. (2006), 'The Intellectual Milieu of Herodotus' in Dewald, C. and Marincola, J. (eds.), *The Cambridge Companion to Herodotus*. Cambridge: Cambridge University Press. 60–75.

Thomas, R. (2000), *Herodotus in Context: Ethnography, Science and the Art of Persuasion*. Cambridge: Cambridge University Press.

Verdenius, W. J. (1966–1967), 'Der Logosbegriff bei Heraklit und Parmenides' in *Phronesis* II; 12. Assen: Van Gorcum. 81–89, 99–117.

Vernant, J. -P. (1983), *Myth and Thought among the Greeks*. London; Boston, MA: Routledge & Kegan Paul.

Wenskus, O. (1982), *Ringkomposition, anaphorisch-rekapitulierende Verbindung und anknüpfende Wiederholung im hippokratischen Corpus*. Frankfurt/Main: R.G. Fischer.

3 Hippocratic *epideixis* and the orality of medical oratory

In the first two chapters, we saw how treatises of the Hippocratic Collection which appear to have been composed for oral delivery to an audience in a sophisticated style should be considered as part of the wider context of Pre-Socratic, Sophistic and some historiographical writing engaged in opening new areas of philosophical enquiry and simultaneously developing new modes of expression. Some of the tensions between and issues raised by the shifts taking place in this period from the authority of verse to the authority of prose and from reliance on oral to more emphasis on written communication were highlighted as part of this background to the emergence of Hippocratic oratory.

We also saw how observations on the content of these works cannot be easily extrapolated from observations on style, and considered the idea that in late fifth-century prose we find examples of authors developing their own approaches to thinking to an extent *through* their use of language. The way in which studies on early scientific and empirical method have at times over-looked the full range of expressive resources late fifth-century authors writing for public display sought to explore and exploit, and tended to establish a dichotomy between form and content, was highlighted and shown to be problematic. We also saw how examples of models of early Greek poetry and prose seeking to present arguments can offer insight into the complexity of Hippocratic oratory as a literary product.

These chapters have aimed to illustrate something of the spirit of the age in which Hippocratic display oratory develops, and draw attention to some of the complexity of approaching this kind of writing, of understanding its nature and purpose. In the following chapters, I seek to consider more closely the question of persuasive function in examples of Hippocratic oratory. What aims might these authors have had in mind? How did their use of language intersect with their conceptual thinking? In what ways does Hippocratic performance prose work to assert authority over its audiences?

In the first and second parts of this chapter, I examine briefly the relevance of the term *epideixis* (ἐπίδειξις) in our understanding of medical display prose, because the five texts I focus on in this study seem most closely to fit this genre and many have been considered examples of *epideixis*. The label *epideixis* implies a range of persuasive functions; it is most closely associated with speeches that seek to praise or blame, with a network of examples of public prose from the late fifth century onwards. I argue below that the term, in its most common definition, is of only limited use in reading Hippocratic display prose. This position is in agreement with recent scholarship on the early history of this term.[1] I argue that some insight can be gained into the earliest notions of 'epideictic' from examining use of this and related terms (i.e. terms which mean 'to show' or 'to display') in examples of performance prose of the Hippocratic Collection.

In the third part of this chapter, I turn to work on the orality of legal oratory in the late fifth century BCE, examining recent scholarship on the orality of oratory, and suggest that oral features of treatises, while they cannot offer con-clusive evidence as to oral dissemination contexts, can offer greater insight into the layers of meaning present in medical texts than has previously been acknowledged. I then offer an analysis of examples of signposting in the five selected Hippocratic treatises and provide further insights into the persuasive aims and functions of these texts.

Epideixis and medical oratory

In the *Rhetoric*, Aristotle classifies persuasive writing into three kinds: judi-cial, epideictic and political (*Rhetoric*, I, 1358a36 f.). This tripartite classifica-tion maintains a gravitational pull on scholars working on early prose writing. Nicole Loraux, for example, in her monumental study of the epideictic funeral oration (of which one of the most famous examples is Pericles' funeral oration as recorded in *On the Peloponnesian War*) in fifth-century Athens, notes that '[Aristotle's] classificatory and normative thought, triumphant in Antiquity, still dominates all modern analyses of the history and function of Greek prose' (Loraux 2006 [1986]: 282–283).[2]

Jouanna's work on the rhetoric of the Hippocratic Collection is no excep-tion to this tendency. In his 1984 article, he seeks to bring Hippocratic display prose within the frame of discussions of early prose writing (seen as specialist, Hippocratic writing has frequently been omitted from such discussions), and does so by referring to Aristotle's taxonomic scheme. He notes that the work of Antiphon and Gorgias' *Defence of Palamedes* are our only examples of judicial speeches in the fifth century; that Gorgias' *Encomium of Helen* and pseudo-Xenophon's *Constitution of Athens,* and [Hippocrates'] *On Breaths* and *On the Art* are our only examples of epideictic work; and that our only example of political speeches comes indirectly through Thucydides (Jouanna 1984: 27). In his work on the rhetoric of Hippocratic display prose, Jouanna consistently employs the term 'epideictic'. He describes *On Breaths* and *On the Art* (Jouanna 1984: 27; cf. Jouanna 1988: 10–29) as epideictic and notes that other 'oral' Hippocratic treatises, for example *On the Sacred Disease*, share certain poetic prose effects common in epideictic speeches (Jouanna 2003: xi).

Furthermore, of the group of 'oral' Hippocratic treatises, established in his 1984 article, Jouanna claims that it is possible to distinguish two parts: 'on the one hand, the oral didactic exposition or "lesson [*cours*]"; on the other hand, the oral epideictic exposition or "speech [*discours*]"' (Jouanna 1984: 32).[3] Following Aristotle in the *Rhetoric*, Jouanna notes that the lesson (*cours*) is characterised by λέξις εἰρομένη ('strung together speech') whereas the speech (*discours*) is characterised by λέξις κατεστραμμένη ('periodic speech') (Jouanna 1984: 36).[4] Jouanna maintains that the only true examples of the oral epideictic exposition – the speech (*discours*) are *On Breaths* and *On the Art* because they end in perorations (typically, enthusiastic or emotional conclusions to speeches) and comments that the main difference between these and the other treatises in the collection is the duration of the oral exposition.[5] Some treatises, which contain elements of '*discours*' are, he claims, designed for lectures in which the author goes into detail and is interested in clarity rather than effect and which take between one hour and ten minutes and one hour and thirty minutes to be delivered. *On Breaths* and *On the Art*, on the other hand, last for around twenty-eight to thirty minutes when delivered (Jouanna 1984: 32–33).

On Breaths and *On the Art* and other 'oral' Hippocratic treatises are viewed as important early examples of *epideixis*, and Aristotle's *Rhetoric* is used by Jouanna as a guide to interpreting the persuasive function of Hippocratic display prose. It is worth considering briefly the status of the term *epideixis* in relation to the Hippocratic Collection.

A key problem with Jouanna's comments is the application of the systematisation of rhetoric by Aristotle (who lived from 384–322 BCE) to material composed in the late fifth century BCE. As argued in the previous chapters, there is no evidence that there was an established and standardised model for explanatory prose writing at this point in history.[6] In his recent edition of the *Rhetoric*, Kennedy notes that Aristotle's definition of epideictic was 'probably only a clarification of existing classifications, seen in the conventions of different genres of Greek oratory' (Kennedy 1991: 46). Kennedy remarks that 'Aristotle . . . thinks of epideictic primarily as funeral oratory or praise of a mythological figure. In such speeches, praise corrects, modifies, or strengthens an audience's belief about the civic virtues or the reputation of an individual' (Kennedy 1991: 47). Furthermore, Aristotle makes no reference in his definition to the genealogy of this genre, and only very few direct references in the rest of *Rhetoric* to examples of what he means by epideictic.[7]

Aristotle's notion of epideictic is narrow compared with the evidence we have for display prose, and his interest is principally in clarifying and categorising existing fourth-century genres, rather than in ascertaining their provenance. Using Aristotle's scheme as a guide to the persuasive function of display prose in the late fifth century is anachronistic and limits our ability to gain a deeper understanding of this important period in the development of prose.

A further problem with Jouanna's use of Aristotle to obtain a sense of possible classifications of Hippocratic texts is that classification only goes a small way to addressing the fraught question of persuasive function. To claim that any given treatise is epideictic only partly answers the question of what the treatise seeks to convey to its audience, in the same way that calling a fictional story in prose a novel merely indicates a set of expectations which the author may or may not conform to or challenge, without identifying the author's aims explicitly.

Paul Demont's chapter on *epideixis*, 'The *Epideixis* (Demonstration) of an Art in the Fifth and Fourth Centuries' (1993) offers a useful analysis of the nature of *epideixis* before Aristotle's time.[8] Demont argues that the term *epideixis* and its cognates are being used in a different and much wider sense in late fifth- and early fourth-century BCE prose, including Hippocratic treatises, than in Aristotle's *Rhetoric* (1993: 181). Unlike Aristotle's other two genres – deliberative and forensic – he claims that the characteristics of epideictic derive from the meaning of the word itself, which is frequently 'to show (something)', a meaning that is also covered by the root verb – *deiknumi* (δείκνυμι) – from which *epideixis* derives (1993: 182). According to Demont, 'In contrast to "*epideixis*", the term "epideictic genre" introduces two special features. Firstly, it is, of course, only an art of rhetorical skill. Secondly, generally the speaker is distinguished from the person whose greatness is praised' (1993: 183).[9] Demont is claiming that in *epideixis*, unlike in Aristotle's epideictic genre, the speaker displays his own art at speaking rather than eulogising somebody else, and notes that there is textual evidence for this kind of speech, unlike Aristotle's genre which indicates a purely oral form.[10]

Demont's study focuses mainly on an aspect of *epideixis* that is not covered in Aristotle's definition, but for which plenty of evidence can be found in the late fifth and early fourth centuries BCE; this is *epideixis* on a *technē*, which can cover any topic from the general to the specialised, and which serves as a demonstration of the excellence or competency of the author (1993: 183). The historical context for this demonstration is the movement of people from one location to another and the consequent need to establish competency and advertise skills to potentially new audiences (1993: 183–184).

Demont notes that the Sophists were probably the first to coin the term *epideixis* to describe public demonstration of oratorical skill and argues that it was this definition and Sophistic demonstration that became most well-known through its depiction in Plato's prestigious works (1993: 184).[11] He argues that the sense of *epideixis* as public demonstration of oratorical skill which came to be promoted by the Sophists and is referred to most clearly in Platonic dialogues is different from *epideixis* as demonstration of technical knowledge. According to Demont, this earlier kind of demonstration of technical knowledge died out as the technical knowledge itself became more established (1993: 187–188). He analyses the demonstrations we find in the Hippocratic Collection that show both the fundamental elements of *epideixis* – theatricality and orality – and which also seek to transmit information, though often information that is more spectacular than useful or accurate, as we see for example in *De articulis*, where fine-looking bandaging techniques are described that had no therapeutic value (1993: 188–190).[12]

The authors of these treatises are, he states, not Sophists but medical practitioners: 'In such lectures, as also in *On the Sacred Disease* and *On the Nature of Human Beings*, the use of these verbs indicates that the expert was present and could prove his abilities and his theories' (1993: 190).[13] The key difference, Demont notes, is that these authors do not seem to be making speeches on *other* topics, as a Sophist would (1993: 191).

In a sense, Demont maintains Aristotle's classificatory instincts, seeking to delimit one kind of author from another, one kind of *epideixis* from another. In *Herodotus in Context*, Rosalind Thomas argues for a greater range and flexibility of meaning in the term than Demont and claims that *epideixis* 'sometimes seems to denote 'display', sometimes a 'display piece' in the sense of a definite genre, and quite often something in-between' (2000: 202). In a more recent chapter (2003) exploring the pragmatics of the relationship between text and performance in the late fifth and early fourth century BCE and the implications of this relationship, Thomas notes the issue of naming and then puts it to one side: 'Whether we call this oral style or epideictic style, or even simply early rhetoric, we seem to be dealing with an identical phenomenon' and

> The early evidence . . . implies that epideictic activity covers a wide range of methods and types of oral discussions, presentations, and speeches, as well as subjects, for in the late fifth century BC it is virtually impossible to separate the epideictic from the agonistic, or the epideixis from oral performance.
>
> (2003: 174)

Thomas' work brings the question of orality back to centre stage of what is meant by *epideixis* in the late fifth-century BCE, though she claims that the evidence provides little indication that the difference between written and spoken versions of performances differed fundamentally in style, noting that written texts tend to reflect oral delivery style:

> The early medical texts confirm that there could be textual differentiation between *epideixeis* and other pieces, with dramatic differences in style and argument between, at one extreme, pieces like *Breaths* and *On the Art*, and *On Regimen* at the other, which is conscious throughout that it is being written, or the *Epidemics*, which include tight lists of data.
>
> (Thomas 2003: 181)

For Thomas, then, an important element of *epideixis* in medical writing is the author's level of involvement with the writing process itself and consciousness of this, in a written form that tends to reflect oral delivery style. For the purposes of this study, given the range of possible meanings and elements associated with *epideixis* in the late fifth century BCE and the issue in some scholarship with the anachronistic application of Aristotle's generic definitions to earlier writing, it is worth considering the evidence that the Hippocratic oratorical texts offer for their persuasive aims and functions.

Also at stake in thinking about *epideixis*, as already noted in the first chapter of this book with the conflicting judgements from Jones and Jouanna about the medical value of treatises such as *On the Art* and *On Breaths* and implied in Demont's comments about regarding *epideixis* as a demonstration of competency, is the extent to which Hippocratic authors engaged in oral exposition of ideas should be considered as belonging to or a challenge to established groups of physicians.[14] In a chapter entitled 'Literacy and the Charlatan in Ancient Greek Medicine', Lesley Dean-Jones argues that, among other things,

> technical medical treatises are amongst the earliest prose works in Greece. Many of these, however, are insufficient for training without oral supplementation, and their appearance is to be explained by the fact that in the fifth century more individuals from non-traditional medical families started to enter the profession and needed aids to mitigate their lack of training from childhood.
>
> (2003: 98)

For Dean-Jones, literacy permits access to previously restricted knowledge and leads some to practice on the basis of book learning alone – these people she identifies as charlatans (2003: 99).

While Dean-Jones' survey of the way in which *iatroi* are referred to before the fourth century BCE, when the first negative portrayals of physicians are shown to appear (2003: 99–108), is convincing evidence of changes to and responses to challenges to the status of medicine towards the end of the fifth century BCE, as the existence of five Hippocratic treatises examined here goes to show, it does not neatly follow that a clear-cut distinction between authorised physician and charlatan existed. Dean-Jones notes that 'The view that there were no charlatans as such in the ancient world rests on the assumption that medical training made little or no difference to an individual's practice and effectiveness as a physician' (2003: 107). In fact, the sense suggested from close examination of medical expository prose is that the very definition of physician and the medical art, as well as the way in which the practise of that art was authorised, was under scrutiny and question. Medicine as an art was undergoing a change that meant that the former distinctions between practitioner and charlatan were unstable and subject to question.

As this book will go on to argue, language use was a key aspect of defining at least some physicians' work, as along with new means of expression came new modes of thinking about medicine and new means of establishing authoritative practice. Dean-Jones' chapter highlights evidence for significant new attitudes to physicians and medicine that arise in the period in which medical ideas began to be written down; however, the chapter underestimates the power of language, treating the rise in literacy as a mere change in communication style, rather than the sign of a more fundamental change in thought processes and underlying concepts. Again, as we saw in the discussion of scholarship on *logos* and style in Chapter 2, a distinction between form and content is assumed which it is problematic to apply to Hippocratic prose writing.

Let us turn, in the next part of this chapter, to a brief analysis of prominent examples of references to 'display' in the Hippocratic texts, to consider how far these can shed further light on notions of exposition at work in individual treatises. Following this, I go on to explore the hallmarks of oral style in medical oratory.

Evidence for Hippocratic notions of display and demonstration

The root meanings of the term *epideixis* (ἐπίδειξις) range from 'showing forth' or 'making known' to 'demonstration' and 'proof'.[15] The *Index Hippocraticus* lists fifteen uses of the terms *epideixis* (ἐπίδειξις) and *epideiknumi* (ἐπιδεικνύμι).[16] As well as these, the *Index* notes other words very closely related to *epideixis* that appear to warrant attention, or at any rate whose exclusion from an examination of the use of *epideixis* cannot obviously be justified within the context of the Hippocratic Collection. These words are given under the entry for the main verb *deiknumi* (δείκνυμι): *apodeiknumi* (ἀποδεικνύμι) (point out, display, make known), *anadeiknum* (ἀναδεικνύμι) (lift up and show, exhibit, display), *endeiknumi* (ἐνδεικνύμι) (mark, point out) and *hupodeiknumi* (ὑποδείκνυμι) (show, indicate) as well as *epideiknumi* (ἐπιδεικνύμι).

As well as *deknumi* (δείκνυμι) and related terms, there are other words, such as *apofainō* (ἀποφαίνω), which could plausibly be included in an investigation into the use of terms meaning broadly 'demonstration' and/or 'display'. The following is a selective discussion of how the term *deiknumi*, with and without any possible prefixes, is being employed in the Hippocratic oratorical treatises, which seeks to ascertain the extent to which a generic notion of *epideixis* is available to or absent from individual treatises.[17]

(a) Use of epideixis in On the Sacred Disease and On Breaths

Let us turn first to the examples of *epideixis* and all related terms in *On the Sacred Disease* and *On Breaths*:

> Εἰ δὲ διὰ τὸ θαυμάσιον θεῖον νομιεῖται, πολλὰ τὰ ἱερὰ νοσήματα ἔσται τούτου εἵνεκεν καὶ οὐχὶ ἕν, ὡς ἐγὼ δείξω ἕτερα οὐδὲν ἧσσον ἐόντα θαυμάσια οὐδὲ τερατώδεα, ἃ οὐδείς νομίζει ἱρὰ εἶναι.

> If it is to be considered divine because it is wonderful, there will be many sacred diseases and not just one, for I will show that other diseases are no less wonderful and portentous, which nobody considers sacred.
>
> (*On the Sacred Disease*, 1.3)

> μετὰ δὲ ταῦτα πρὸς αὐτὰ τὰ ἔργα τῷ αὐτῷ λόγῳ πορευθεὶς ἐπιδείξω τὰ νοσήματα τούτου ἀπόγονά τε καὶ ἔκγονα πάντα ἐόντα.

> after this I will by the same reasoning proceed to the physical evidence and I will show that all diseases come about from things coming to and leaving the body.
>
> (*On Breaths*, 5.2)

In the first example, from *On the Sacred Disease*, the author announces what he is about to offer to his audience; the term 'δείκνυμι' 'I show' used in the passage above in the first person of the future, with its grammatical objects, serves as an advertisement to attract the attention of the audience (live or otherwise) and as a structural device to make clear the subject of the treatise. The use of the first person is striking, suggesting emphasis on the identity of the speaker as much as on the subject of the treatise. The sense that this verb is used as a boast or a dramatic claim is derived from the contrast made between the speaker's stated understanding of the issue and that of everybody else ('οὐδείς' 'nobody [else]'). In the second example, from near the beginning of *On Breaths*, we find the term used in a similar fashion: in the first person future, with an announcement as to what is to follow in the treatise and in the form of a grand claim to be able to show the cause of all diseases.

The next two examples are taken from the final section of *On Breaths*:

Φαίνονται τοίνυν αἱ φῦσαι διὰ πάντων τούτων μάλιστα πολυπρηγμονέουσαι . . . Τὸ δὲ αἴτιον τῶν νούσων ἐὸν τοῦτο ἐπιδέδεικταί μοι.

So it is clear therefore that breaths are the most active agents in all these things . . . that breaths are the cause of diseases has been shown by me.

(*On Breaths*, 15.1)

Ἐπέδειξα δὲ τὸ πνεῦμα καὶ ἐν τοῖσιν ὅλοισι πρήγμασι δυναστεῦον καὶ ἐν τοῖσι σώμασι τῶν ζῴων.

I have shown that air exercises its power in the universe and in the bodies of living beings.

(*On Breaths*, 15.2)

Here, the author announces again what the subject of his treatise has been. Although they appear in the final section of the treatise, these are not concluding remarks in the sense that they summarise what has been said by the author; rather they almost repeat the claim made at the beginning of the treatise (above), only stating here explicitly that what is meant by 'things coming to and leaving the body' is air. Again, the claims are either in the first person of the verb, or specify the author using the dative of the agent. The claims are also emphatic and direct because they are so general and because they imply a definitive conclusion.

The one further use of a term related to *epideixis* in *On the Sacred Disease* does not appear in a similar context to those above and does not refer to the treatise itself nor to the author of the treatise. Nevertheless, it can also offer insight into what is understood by *epideixis* in the sense of an oral presentation.

Τὰ γοῦν μέγιστα τῶν ἁμαρτημάτων καὶ ἀνοσιώτατα τὸ θεῖόν ἐστι τὸ καθαῖρον καὶ ἁγνίζον καὶ ῥύμμα γινόμενον ἡμῖν· αὐτοί τε ὅρους τοῖσι θεοῖσι τῶν ἱρῶν καὶ τῶν τεμενέων ἀποδείκνυμεν, ὡς ἂν μηδεὶς ὑπερβαίνῃ ἢν μὴ ἁγνεύῃ, εἰσιόντες τε ἡμεῖς περιρραινόμεθα οὐχ ὡς μιαινόμενοι, ἀλλ' ‘εἴ τι καὶ πρότερον ἔχομεν μύσος, τοῦτο ἀφαγνιούμενοι.

At any rate, it is the divine that is the purifier, the sanctifier and the cleanser of the greatest and most impious of our transgressions; and we ourselves establish boundaries to the sanctuaries and precincts of the gods, so that nobody may cross them unless pure; and when we enter we sprinkle ourselves, not so as to make ourselves impure, but in order to wash away any pollution we may have already contracted.

(*On the Sacred Disease*, 1.13)

The verb *apodeiknumen* (ἀποδείκνυμεν) here refers to the action of setting up or marking out (in this case) physical boundaries ('ὅρους') around sacred spaces so as to distinguish sacred from non-sacred space. This time we have a participle form in the first person plural, and the verb refers to a general custom. The use of this term connects with other uses of the term in that the fundamental sense is one of making something clear to people and also of establishing an authority. The sense of defining territory gives us a hint of the agonistic context of oral presentation in which this same term is also used. There is also a direct connection between the demarcation of physical space in the temple and the definition in the argument of the treatise in that both the temple boundary and the author's exposition seek to define what is and is not sacred.[18]

The uses of *epideixis* in *On the Sacred Disease* and *On Breaths* give the impression that the word is used for announcing a display of knowledge, often alongside dramatic or emphatic claims that would attract attention and in the first person, suggesting that the identity of the speaker is important in such contexts. The use of *apodeixis* in *On the Sacred Disease* indicates the public marking of boundaries and analogously hints at the establishment of authority by speakers and the agonistic context of display. Broadly, this fits with the notion of the genre or characteristic style of *epideixis* discussed in the previous chapter. It also seems to confirm a distinction in meaning between the terms *apodeixis* and *epideixis*. Further examples of the use of these terms in other Hippocratic treatises corroborate this evidence, but what we also find is evidence that these terms were being used in a way which was rather novel and that their reference to a specific genre or style in this period is tentative and in the process of being defined. They are related to the subject matter being discussed and are malleable according to the context in which they are deployed.

(b) Epideixis *and* apodeixis *in* On the Art *and* On the Nature of Human Beings

Near the beginning of *On the Art*, we find the following:

Περὶ μὲν οὖν τούτων εἴ γέ τις μὴ ἱκανῶς ἐκ τῶν εἰρημένων σύνίησιν, ἐν ἄλλοισιν ἂν λόγοισι σαφέστερον διδαχθείη· περὶ δὲ ἰητρικῆς – ἐς ταύτην γὰρ ὁ λόγος –, ταύτης οὖν τὴν ἀπόδειξιν ποιήσομαι. Καὶ πρῶτόν γε διοριεῦμαι ὃ νομίζω ἰητρικὴν εἶναι· τὸ δὴ πάμπαν ἀπαλλάσσειν τῶν νοσεόντων τοὺς καμάτους καὶ τῶν νοσημάτων τὰς σφοδρότητας ἀμβλύνειν, καὶ τὸ μὴ ἐγχειρεῖν τοῖσι κεκρατημένοισιν ὑπὸ τῶν νοσημάτων, εἰδότας ὅτι πάντα ταῦτα δύναται ἰητρική. Ὡς οὖν ποιεῖ τε ταῦτα καὶ οἵη τέ ἐστιν διὰ παντὸς ποιεῖν, περὶ τούτου μοι ὁ λοιπὸς λόγος ἤδη ἔσται· Ἐν δὲ τῇ τῆς τέχνης ἀποδείξει ἅμα καὶ τοὺς λόγους τῶν αἰσχύνειν αὐτὴν οἰομένων ἀναιρήσω, ᾗ ἂν ἕκαστος αὐτῶν πρήσσειν τι οἰόμενος τυγχάνῃ.

Concerning the preceding questions, if anyone has not sufficiently under-stood what has been said, a clearer explanation can be found more in other treatises. As for medicine – for this is the subject of this treatise – I will make a demonstration of it. First, I will define what I think medicine is. It is to relieve the sick completely from their suffering, and to dull the most violent of illnesses, and not to treat those who are completely over-powered by disease, knowing that medicine is able to do all the things above. In the rest of my treatise, I will establish that medicine does these things and that it is able to do so in all circumstances. At the same time as making a demonstration of the existence of the art, I will destroy the arguments of those who think to shame it, and I will challenge them on the points where each of them believes he has made some discovery.

(*On the Art*, 3.1–3)

The author states in this extract that he will 'produce a demonstration of medi-cine'. The context is of a discussion of the existence of arts (τέχναι) in Section 2 of the treatise. In this section, the author has argued that all arts correspond to a reality and that in effect what is non-existent by definition cannot be discussed:

τὰ μὲν ἐόντα αἰεὶ ὁρᾶταί τε καὶ γινώσκεται, τὰ δὲ μὴ ἐόντα οὔτε ὁρᾶται οὔτε γινώσκεται. Γινώσκεται τοίνυν δεδειγμένων ἤδη τῶν τεχνέων, καὶ οὐδεμία ἐστὶν ἥ γε ἔκ τινος εἴδεος οὐχ ὁρᾶται.

Whatever exists is always seen and known; whatever does not exist is neither seen nor known. They are known, then, on the basis of the prior demonstration of [the existence of] the arts, and there is no art which is not seen from some [really existing] form.

(*On the Art*, 2.2)

Given this context, the demonstration referred to in the excerpt above appears to be an introduction to the art of medicine or an exposition of what must, because it can be known, be the case about medicine. The author's use of the noun *apodeixis* (ἀπόδειξις) in the passage above coupled with the verb 'ποιήσομαι' 'I will make' suggests a defined activity of exposition.[19] The definite article used alongside this – 'τὴν ἀπόδειξιν' 'a / the demonstration' – suggests that the author's exposition will aim to be definitive. The term *apodeixis* as a definitive activity reflects the context in which it is being used: the author is aiming at a solid and fundamental defence of the art of medicine since the very existence of the art of medicine is at stake here.

The author uses the term *logos* (λόγος) in the above to refer to his own work as well as *apodeixis*: he switches from referring to the treatise as a whole with the term *logos* to outlining the contents of his exposition of medicine with the term *apodeixis*, suggesting that the latter is more specific to the expository, defensive role of the treatise and the former is more general. *Apodeixis* in this passage seems to convey an unquestionably authoritative or positive account or set of arguments as part of a competitive context. The word hints at an epistemological position that connects demonstration with knowledge and the existence of the art of medicine with the possibility of its demonstration.[20]

In *On the Nature of Human Beings* we find the author giving a breakdown of what he means by the term *apodeixis*:

> ταὐτὰ δὲ λέγω ταῦτα καὶ περὶ τοῦ φάσκοντος φλέγμα εἶναι τὸν ἄνθρωπον, καὶ περὶ τοῦ χολὴν φάσκοντος εἶναι. ἐγὼ μὲν γὰρ ἀποδείξω ἃ ἂν φήσω τὸν ἄνθρωπον εἶναι, καὶ κατὰ [τὸν] νόμον καὶ κατὰ [τὴν] φύσιν, ἀεὶ ταὐτὰ ἐόντα ὁμοίως, καὶ νέου ἐόντος καὶ γέροντος, καὶ τῆς ὥρης ψυχρῆς ἐούσης καὶ θερμῆς, καὶ τεκμήρια παρέξω, καὶ ἀνάγκας ἀποφανέω, δι᾽ ἃς ἕκαστον αὔξεταί τε καὶ φθίνει ἐν τῷ σώματι.

> I make the same remarks concerning those who claim that the human is only phlegm and those who claim that it is only bile. So, I will demonstrate that those elements both according to custom and according to nature which I claim the human to consist of are constantly and invariably the same, in youth and in old age, and in the cold and hot season; and I will provide signs and show the compelling factors through which each element grows and diminishes in the body.
>
> (*On the Nature of Human Beings*, 2.4–5)

In this extract, we find 'ἀποδείξω' 'I will demonstrate' used in the first person singular of the future at the beginning of the treatise, advertising the author and his account and announcing what is to follow as was the case with the use of 'ἐπιδείξω' 'I will show' in *On the Sacred Disease* and *On Breaths* above.

The author also states that he will give an account of what he says human beings are like – 'Ἐγὼ μὲν γὰρ ἀποδείξω, ἃ ἂν φήσω τὸν ἄνθρωπον εἶναι' 'I will demonstrate that those elements which I claim the human to consist of' – giving the impression of distinction between a statement and supporting explanation.[21] The author also points out different components of his account: 'τεκμήρια παρέξω' 'I will provide evidence' and 'ἀνάγκας ἀποφανῶ' I will show proofs/necessary connections'. The fact that the author announces his notion of demonstration suggests that it would not have been self-evident to his audience what a demonstration consisted of, and that it could contain different components. The author is both giving an explanation and announcing to his audience what an explanation consists of.

In both *On the Art* and *On the Nature of Human Beings* we gain the sense of *apodeixis* as a definitive account which fits in with the notion of the term referring to a particular style or genre; in subtly different ways, however, the authors of both treatises also seek to indicate this definitiveness, implying that it was not self-evident and that the term refers to a type of account that was in the process of being shaped and established.

Similar to the way that statement and explanation are being distinguished in *On the Nature of Human Beings*, the author of *On Ancient Medicine* writes:

> Ὅστις δὲ ταῦτα ἀποβαλὼν καὶ ἀποδοκιμάσας πάντα ἑτέρῃ ὁδῷ καὶ ἑτέρῳ σχήματι ἐπιχειρεῖ ζητεῖν καί φησί ἐξευρηκέναι, ἐξηπάτηται καὶ ἐξαπατᾶται· ἀδύνατον γάρ. Δι’ ἃς δὲ ἀνάγκας ἀδύνατον ἐγὼ πειρήσομαι ἐπιδεῖξαι λέγων καὶ ἐπιδεικνύων τὴν τέχνην ὅ τι ἐστίν.

> But anyone who, casting aside and rejecting all these means, attempts to conduct research in any other way or after another fashion, and asserts that he has found out anything, is and has been the victim of deception. His assertion is impossible; the causes of its impossibility I will endeavour to expound by a statement and exposition of what the art is.
>
> (*On Ancient Medicine*, 2.2)

Here the term 'λέγων' 'saying' is used alongside 'ἐπιδεικνύων' 'demonstrating', recalling the use of 'φημί' 'I say' alongside 'ἀποδείκνυμι' 'I demonstrate' in *On the Nature of Human Beings* quoted above. *Epideixis* here is described as discussing necessary relationships – 'ἀνάγκας' 'proofs / necessary connections' – and a definitive position – 'ἀδύνατον' '– and it is implied that it may involve effort and may not be successful – 'πειρήσομαι' 'I will try'. 'λέγων' 'saying' may or may not be part of this demonstration depending on whether it is read as in contrast to or somehow connected with *epideixis* in the phrase 'λέγων καὶ ἐπιδεικνύων' 'saying and demonstrating'; either way it is the word *epideixis* that is more precisely accounted for here, suggesting that it is a more specific term for this author, yet still one that requires qualification.

(c) Evidence for visual and non-verbal notions of epideixis

The impression that the term *epideixis* was not used in the context of the 'oral' treatises of the Hippocratic Collection with a self-evident meaning, can be reinforced with evidence from *On the Art* which introduces the possibility of different formats for *epideixis*:

Ὅτι μὲν οὖν καὶ λόγους ἐν ἑωυτῇ εὐπόρους ἐς τὰς ἐπικουρίας ἔχει ἡ ἰητρικὴ καὶ οὐκ εὐδιορθώτοισι δικαίως οὐκ ἂν ἐγχειρέοι τῇσι νούσοισιν ἢ ἐγχειρευμένας ἀναμαρτήτους ἂν παρέχοι, οἵ τε νῦν λεγόμενοι λόγοι δηλοῦσιν αἵ τε τῶν εἰδότων τὴν τέχνην ἐπιδείξιες, ἃς ἐκ τῶν ἔργων ἥδιον ἢ ἐκ τῶν λόγων ἐπιδεικνύουσιν, οὐ τὸ λέγειν καταμελετήσαντες, ἀλλὰ τὴν πίστιν τῷ πλήθει, ἐξ ὧν ἂν ἴδωσιν, οἰκειοτέρην ἡγεύμενοι ἢ ἐξ ὧν ἂν ἀκούσωσιν.

Now that medicine in itself has arguments full of resources for its treatments, and that it would rightly refuse to undertake problematic cases, or undertaking them would do so without making a mistake, is shown both by arguments now being given and by the demonstrations of those versed in the art, demonstrations which are given more readily through action than through words, and not by attention to words, under the belief that the multitude find it more natural to be convinced by what they have seen than what they have heard.

(*On the Art*, 13.1)

Here, the author refers to his own treatise in terms of a series of arguments 'οἵ . . . λεγόμενοι λόγοι' '[the] arguments now being given' which is parallel to 'αἵ . . . τῶν εἰδότων τὴν τέχνην ἐπιδείξιες' 'the demonstrations of those versed in the art'. However, in this treatise the demonstrations referred to in the latter quotation are said to be given 'ἐκ τῶν ἔργων ἥδιον ἢ ἐκ τῶν λόγων ἐπιδεικνύουσιν 'more readily through action than through words' and this in response to the perceived requirements of persuading a crowd of listeners. This passage hints at a world of practical demonstrations before crowds and therefore suggests a closer analogy with theatre than simply spoken explanations. In this passage the term *epideixis* refers to visual elements of demonstration that we have very little evidence for, thus supporting the idea that the term and the phenomena it referred to were in the process of being established when this treatise was written.

The visual element to *epideixis* is also hinted at in this passage from *On Ancient Medicine*, which describes the body giving visual signs of internal disorder:

Τὰ δ' ἄλλα πάντα περὶ τὸν ἄνθρωπον, ὅσῳ ἂν πλείοσι μίσγηται, τοσούτῳ ἠπιώτερα καὶ βελτίονα. Πάντων δ' ἄριστα διάκειται ὤνθρωπος, ὅταν πέσσηται καὶ ἐν ἡσυχίῃ ᾖ μηδεμίαν δύναμιν ἰδίην ἀποδεικνύμενα. Περὶ μὲν οὖν τούτων ἱκανῶς μοι ἡγεῦμαι ἐπιδεδεῖχθαι.

But all other components of a human become milder and better the greater the number of other components with which they are mixed. A human is in the best possible condition when there is complete coction and calm, with no particular power displayed. I think that I have explained this subject sufficiently.

(*On Ancient Medicine*, 19.7–20.1)

This is taken from the second part of *On Ancient Medicine*, in which the author challenges those who claim that hot, cold, dry and wet are the essential powers of the human being (15.1 f). He claims that these people have never discovered these powers acting purely – that is, not mixed with other qualities – and that they have the same range of foodstuffs available for use as remedies as anybody else, noting that they are not able to ascribe to these foodstuffs a single power (for example, cold) but rather that they claim that they always have a mixed power (for example, cold *and* bitter) (15.2–4) The author then argues through a number of examples of common situations involving temperature changes in the body that hot and cold cannot in fact be considered strong powers in the body since when they are intermingled they cause no trouble, and when one does become more powerful than the other, they quickly return to a balanced state (16. 1–6). In cases of fever, the author states, it is not heat but some other quality that is the main cause of the fever (16.7–17.3).

The author then discusses different causes of coryza (that is, nasal congestion, a symptom of the common cold), including cases in which cold is the only cause (contradicting his earlier claim that the four powers first mentioned do not act independently) (*On Ancient Medicine*, 18.1–4). Mixing and coction are necessary, he claims, to remedy those cases that are caused by acrimony and *crasis* among the humours, but not for those caused by cold alone. A few other cases of illness derived from hot or cold are then listed, before the author states that all the rest result from qualities rather than powers (19.1–6). The author then ends this section by noting that the elements of the body are least troublesome when mixed – adding that hot can only mix with cold and vice versa (19.7).

The passage quoted directly above concludes this section by stating that the highest form of health is obtained when no one power becomes dominant. Here the author uses the term 'ἀποδεικνύμενος' meaning 'shows itself' referring to the powers just mentioned, such as discharge from the nose. There is an analogy with the sense of 'ἐπιδεδεῖχθαι' 'to have explained' used in the following line: on the one hand the body makes external signals as to its internal state and on the other hand the author proclaims his ideas to make public his thoughts to his audience.

As elsewhere, it is significant that these terms come at the end of a passage of explanation; the author steps back from the act of explanation to underline what has been going on and close off this section of his treatise and, analogously, he moves from discussing the internal processes of the body to external signs. These two uses of *deknumi* close together in the treatise then add to other hints we have seen of a sense of revelation to a public, and of making the largely unseen seen, which can be understood in both a visual and a verbal sense.

There are also examples of the use of *deiknumi* that do not clearly refer to either a verbal or a practical demonstration:

Ἔτι δὲ καὶ ἐν τοῖσιν ἀσάρκοισι τοιαύτη ἔνεστιν οἵη καὶ ἐν τοῖσιν εὐσάρκοισιν ἐνεῖναι δέδεικται.

Furthermore, there exists on the parts where flesh is absent a cavity sim-ilar to the one whose existence has been demonstrated for the parts cov-ered in flesh.

(On the Art, 10.4)

The demonstration referred to here may refer to the explanation given directly prior to this passage in the treatise, or it could equally or additionally suggest that the author may make his point by indicating the features mentioned on a model.

In this discussion, we have gained some insight into the use of the term *epideixis* at the level of individual examples from 'oral' treatises of the Hip-pocratic Collection. We have seen that while the term does normally refer to an account or explanation as opposed to a statement, corroborating Demont's and Thomas' analyses, there is also evidence that it was necessary for these authors to spell out the meaning of the term and that it may have also served a persuasive purpose in establishing an author's authority. Furthermore, we have seen evidence that the term cannot easily be limited to a verbal genre or style since it can refer to visual or physical demonstration, of which we have very little evidence. This again emphasises the stretch of this term and pro-vides further support for the sense that it was in the process of being defined in this period.

The orality of Hippocratic oratorical texts

If the use of the term 'δείκνυμι' 'to show' and related words in the Hippocratic oratorical treatises shows a wide range of notions of revelation and display in different formats, we should also consider the reason why these authors elect to make claims about the aims and intentions of their work in the first place. In this last section of the chapter, I examine the presence of claims to display or demonstrate from another angle, as part of a range of features of oral style. To do this, I turn first to a chapter by Michael Gagarin on the orality of oratory which sets out some of the groundwork for the discussion to follow.

In the chapter, an addition to the relatively limited scholarship on the oral nature of oratory, Gagarin argues that 'there are clear differences between oratory to be read and oratory written to be performed orally and that these differences are related to oral performance' (1998: 164).[22] He compares the *Second Tetralogy* of Antiphon, the originator of forensic logography, with Gorgias' *Encomium of Helen*, the work of the most prominent Sophistic orator.

This work on the differences between oratory composed for performance and oratory composed to be read is a useful point of reference which can be used to take us a step forward from verbal references to display in Hippocratic writing to identification and analysis of specific persuasive features that are hallmarks of oratory and help shed further light on the question of persuasive function of Hippocratic display prose. Gagarin provides a framework for thinking more deeply about whether any given work of presumed oratory was composed for oral performance and the extent to which this may be reflected in features of the writing.

In the chapter, Gagarin contrasts a speech which is composed primarily to be delivered orally – Gorgias' *Encomium of Helen*, a mock defence of Helen of Troy against the charge that she initiated the Trojan War – with an example of a speech which he argues was composed primarily for a reading public: the defendant's first speech in Antiphon's *Second Tetralogy*, a prosecution for accidental homicide which is dated to the late fifth, early fourth century (see Gagarin 1997).[23] Gagarin argues that

> Among the features of oral style we can identify in *Helen* are signposts, ring composition, parallelism, parataxis, simplified sentence structure, and, of course, the notorious 'Gorgianic' verbal effects. Antiphon, by contrast, builds his argument largely without these features: he does not alert the reader where he is going, and he uses a more complex syntax, heavily dependent on participles, with very little verbal assonance.
>
> (1998: 168)

He also notes that 'Antiphon presents a radically new argument supported by generalisation and analysis, whereas Gorgias' basic argument is less innovative and he avoids analysis or generalisations even when it suggests itself' (1998: 168).

To be clear, these features are (1) signposts, which are phrases or words that alert the listener to the stage of progression within the speech and make explicit reference to its structure; (2) ring composition, whereby the structure moves out from a starting point and back to the same starting point; (3) parallelism and use of parataxis, by which is meant the use of sentences or parts of sentences which mirror one another or which complement one another;[24] (4) antitheses, which Gagarin notes are usually brief in *Helen* and are longer, involve more complex ideas and are sometimes combined into complex clusters in the extract from the *Tetralogies*; (5) word order: Gagarin notes Antiphon's tendency towards extreme hyperbaton – that is, rearrangement of customary word order, and Gorgias' tendency only towards a mild version of this; (6) sentence length, with Antiphon's sentences significantly – around a third – longer than Gorgias'; (7) verbal effects, which Gagarin notes Antiphon generally avoids, while Gorgias famously embraces (1998: 168–171).

As well as these stylistic features, which characterise Gorgias' 'oral' oratory in contrast with Antiphon's oratory to be read, Gagarin notes that 'Antiphon presents a radically new argument supported by generalisation and analysis, whereas Gorgias' basic argument is less innovative and he avoids analysis or generalisation even when it suggests itself' (1998: 168), thus adding three further features, more of content than of style, to consider in comparing these speeches: (1) innovation, (2) generalisation and (3) analysis.

In discussing Antiphon's legal speeches and an extant example of Gorgias' work, Gagarin brings out a stark contrast between what he claims is clear and simple oratory to be heard and more complex oratory to be read: 'Although these stylistic differences may be more a matter of degree than kind, taken together they form a clear contrast between clarity and simplicity on the one hand and complexity, even obscurity, on the other' (1998: 171).

However, while the stylistic differences that Gagarin highlights are clearly indicative of major differences between the sources he contrasts, these are not necessarily to be attributed to different forms of dissemination. Antiphon and Gorgias are writing for very different purposes – Antiphon's legal speeches seem to have been used for real cases in court while Gorgias' *Helen* is clearly an imaginative play on the genre of legal defence. The assumption that Gagarin makes is that form is indicative only of persuasive context; yet, it may also be indicative of and closely intersect with theoretical content. The whimsy and humour of Gorgias' display are powerfully communicated by a form of language that is reflexive and replete with repetition and simplicity: Gorgias' *Helen* is a child-like legal defence, but that does not mean that it was necessarily intended as a certain form of communication. It could easily suit both a performance before a crowd, and a textbook-style model of speech composition. Similarly, it is not surprising that Antiphon's legal speeches are more complex in compositional techniques given the gravity and complexity of content that they seek to communicate: they could be suitable for oral dissemination, or private reading, or both.

Gagarin does usefully identify stylistic features which are important to these authors, and which are being exploited for persuasive effect. The difficulty comes in how far these effects can be judged to indicate a certain communicative context, how far they merely reflect a certain context and how far they are being put to service in conjunction with theoretical content: these are questions that Gagarin does not broach in his chapter.

In the next chapter of this study, on sound in Hippocratic display oratory, I will consider the use of what Gagarin terms 'verbal effects', identified here as a hallmark of 'oral' prose, and consider the persuasive function of these features. In Chapter 5, I will consider the use of antitheses, again with a view to uncovering the persuasive and communicative potential of this feature. I argue that while these clearly are persuasive features related to a culture attuned to oral display oratory, their use does not translate neatly into a picture of whether any given treatise was primarily composed for one context or another; indeed, I suggest that it would be futile to try to claim that any text is exclusively used for one purpose or another.

Before moving on to do this, and to lead into the discussion in the following two chapters, it is worthwhile to illustrate an example of my approach by considering in further detail claims to display and demonstration already touched on above as signposting features characteristic of 'oral' texts. In the section above, we saw that all five selected Hippocratic display prose texts made reference to demonstration in the form of an announcement or promise to the audience about what will be demonstrated. The most emphatic references to display were found in *On Ancient Medicine*, *On the Art* and *On Breaths*, though all five treatises indicated an intention to make a demonstration. Is there, then, a sense that because of the evidence of emphasis on signposting these three Hippocratic treatises are more deliberately designed for an oral dissemination context than *On the Sacred Disease* and *On the Nature of Human Beings*? I suggest below that while we do find differences in the way signposting is being used, this cannot simply indicate persuasive context: the issues at stake are more complex than this, though there *are* hints as to persuasive context in places.

(a) On the Art

We find many examples of signposting in this treatise, although it is not consistently present throughout. For example, the following extract, in which the author announces the intention for his treatise:

> Περὶ μὲν οὖν τούτων εἴ γέ τις μὴ ἱκανῶς ἐκ τῶν εἰρημένων ξύνίησιν, ἐν ἄλλοισιν ἂν λόγοισιν σαφέστερον διδαχθεή· περὶ δὲ ἰητρικῆς – ἐς ταύτην γὰρ ὁ λόγος –, ταύτης οὖν τὴν ἀπόδειξιν ποιήσομαι.

> Concerning on the one hand these matters, then, should anyone not have reached a sufficient understanding from what has been said, clearer instruction may be given in other discourses. Concerning on the other

hand medicine – as this is the subject of this discourse – about this, then, I will now give a demonstration.

(3.1)

This sentence serves to move the discussion on from the opening general statements about the existence of arts in general to the existence and defence of the art of medicine. There is more than a simple indication of what is to come: the author is also seeking to manage the expectations of the audience or reader and indicate closure on the topic of art (τέχνη) in general. The signpost is emphatic in the sense that it brings one topic to a close, redirecting to other treatises for further information, stating the main topic of the treatise and announcing the intention of the author. The balancing phrasing – 'Περὶ μὲν . . . περὶ δὲ' 'concerning on the one hand . . . concerning on the other hand' – also builds an antithesis into the signpost and we find parallelism in the repeated reference to the subject 'ἰητρικῆς . . . ταύτην . . . ταύτης' 'medicine . . . this . . . this'.

On this account alone, the treatise would seem to be designed for oral dissemination, following Gagarin's analysis. Yet, this could equally be an example of an author taking constructions which emerge most prominently from oral discussion contexts and committing them to the page. There is attention to sound and to rhythm as we might expect from the spoken word, but no conclusive evidence about performance context. We *can*, however, note a certain intimacy of relation between the author and reader or audience, and a use of language which is influenced by attention to its sound.

(b) On the Sacred Disease

There is very little signposting in this treatise beyond basic statements of topic, as at the beginning of the treatise:

Περὶ τῆς ἱερῆς νούσου καλεομένης ὧδ' ἔχει . . .

This is how things are concerning the disease called sacred . . .

(On the Sacred Disease, 1.1)

However, topic statements are repeated at the beginning of Sections 1 and 2 and are strategically placed to help structure the treatise. As we saw with the reference to display above (pages 63–5), the author's indications of structure are brief and succinct, with precise detail of subject matter included and prominent.

In contrast to the quotation from *On the Art* above, this signpost includes no first-person verb, no parallelism, no antithetical constructions. Based on this limited evidence alone, *On the Sacred Disease* is likely to have been composed for a somewhat different context from *On the Art*. It is possible that this is a context in which the treatise is read silently or quietly by an individual. But it is also possible that this was written for dissemination before a group of physicians learning about the disease. The use of phonic features is less prominent than in *On the Art*, but again this does not necessarily translate into evidence for dissemination context. It does indicate an author apparently less engaged with sound than the author of *On the Art*; yet, as I argue below, there is significant engagement of antithetical constructions in this treatise.

(c) On Ancient Medicine

In the references to display in *On Ancient Medicine* above, we saw emphatic and specific references to what the author intended to demonstrate. There are more, and more elaborate examples of signposting than in *On the Sacred Disease*. As with the references to demonstration above, the signposts tend to be succinct and precise.

> Ἐπὶ δὲ τῶν τὸν καινὸν τρόπον τὴν τέχνην ζητεύντων ἐξ ὑποθέσιος λόγον ἐπανελθεῖν βούλομαι.

> But I wish to return to the account of those who pursue their researches in the art according to the new method, from a hypothesis.
>
> (*On Ancient Medicine*, 13.1)

This example of signposting indicates a shift and return from the discussion of the original discovery of medicine through trial and error – the 'archaeology' of medicine –, which occupies Sections 2–12 of the treatise, to criticism of the medical innovators which occupies the opening of the treatise, Sections 1–2 and Sections 13–19.

Other examples of signposting in the treatise are more informal in tone, loosely indicating what has been said and what is to come rather than stipulating intent, as in the following, for instance:

> Περὶ δὲ δυναμίων, χυμῶν αὐτῶν τε ἕκαστος ὅ τι δύναται ποιεῖν τὸν ἄνθρωπον ἐσκέφθαι, ὥσπερ καὶ πρότερον εἴρηται, καὶ τὴν συγγένειαν ὡς ἔχουσι πρὸς ἀλλήλους. Λέγω δὲ τὸ τοιοῦτον.

> Concerning powers, it is necessary to examine both what each one of the humours in itself is able to do to the human being, as has already been said, and also their kinship with one another. I mean something like the following.
>
> (*On Ancient Medicine*, 24.1)

Broadly, we find in these examples the sense of an author aiming to communicate a message as clearly as possible to an audience, and explicitly acknowledging this as his intention. As with the phrase 'πειρήσομαι ἐπιδεῖξαι, λέγων καὶ ἐπιδεικνύων τὴν τέχνην ὅτι ἐστίν' 'I will endeavour to expound [this] by a statement and exposition of what the art is' cited above (2.2) the signposting is specific and detailed.

Like *On the Art* and unlike *On the Sacred Disease* the author refers clearly to his intentions using a first-person verb with reference to the subject of the treatise. The reference here to speaking certainly suggests that the treatise was read out in some form; this could be a script for a lecture or a record of a lecture, or merely a colloquial use of the verb 'to speak' in a period when distinctions between written and oral were shifting.

(d) On the Nature of Human Beings

This treatise shows continual use of signposting, particularly in the first two-thirds of the treatise. For example:

> ἐγὼ μὲν γὰρ ἀποδείξω, ἃ ἂν φήσω τὸν ἄνθρωπον εἶναι, καὶ κατὰ τὸν νόμον καὶ κατὰ τὴν φύσιν, ἀεὶ τὰ αὐτὰ ἐόντα ὁμοίως, καὶ νέου ἐόντος καὶ γέροντος, καὶ τῆς ὥρης ψυχρῆς ἐούσης καὶ θερμῆς, καὶ τεκμήρια παρέξω, καὶ ἀνάγκας ἀποφανῶ, δι᾽ ἃς ἕκαστον αὔξεταί τε καὶ φθίνει ἐν τῷ σώματι.

> I for my part will prove that what I declare to be the constituents of a human are, according to both convention and nature, always alike the same; it makes no difference whether the man be young or old, or whether the season be cold or hot. I will also bring evidence, and set forth the necessary causes why each constituent grows or decreases in the body.
>
> (*On the Nature of Human Beings*, 2.5)

Here the author announces the nature and focus of the discussion to follow and indicates key features of this discussion (evidence, consideration of causes). There is a sense of promise to the listener or reader in this signpost, which we do not find in the examples from the other four treatises: we have a claim which the author announces will be supported with demonstration. First-person signposting verbs in the future tense are used near the beginning of *On the Art* ('τὴν ἀπόδειξιν ποιήσομαι' 'I will give a demonstration' (3.1)) and *On Ancient Medicine* ('πειρήσομαι ἐπιδεῖξαι' 'I will try to demonstrate' (2.2)), and with more certainty and less suspense in *On the Sacred Disease* ('ἐγὼ δείξω' 'I will show' (1.3)). The claim 'ἐγὼ μὲν γὰρ ἀποδείξω, ἃ ἂν φήσω . . . εἶναι . . ' 'I will demonstrate what I declare . . . to be . . . ' may simply be a variation on these examples and a standard feature of the opening of extended prose treatises. There is a sense, however, in the drawn-out syntax and of repetition of first-person verb of a greater degree emphasis on display. A very similar construction is used earlier in the treatise:

> Εἰπὼν δέ, ἃ ἂν φήσω τὸν ἄνθρωπον εἶναι, ἀποφανεῖν αἰεὶ ταὐτὰ ἐόντα καὶ κατὰ νόμον καὶ κατὰ φύσιν, φημὶ δὲ εἶναι αἷμα καὶ φλέγμα καὶ χολὴν ξανθὴν καὶ μέλαιναν.

> Now I promised to show that what are according to me the constituents of humans remain always the same, according to both convention and nature, so I declare that the constituents are blood, phlegm, yellow bile and black bile.

> *(On the Nature of Human Beings*, 5.1)

There is certainly a sense of signposting being in this treatise to build a sense of intention emphatically and by referring to fulfilment of a promise, to engage emotionally with the audience, as well as to structure the treatise. As with the examples above, however, this need not necessarily be in an exclusively oral or quiet/silent-reading context and seems likely to have been used for both. The references to speaking and seeing do reflect oral habits, but do not provide strong evidence for an 'oral' text: after all, the source we study is written.

(e) On Breaths

The treatise displays continuous and consistent use of signposting, as, for example:

> Ὅτι μὲν οὖν μεγάλη κοινωνίη ἅπασι τοῖσι ζῴοισι τοῦ ἠέρος ἐστίν, εἴρηται· μετὰ τοῦτο τοίνυν ῥητέον, ὡς οὐκ ἄλλοθέν ποθεν εἰκός ἐστι γίνεσθαι τὰς ἀρρωστίας ἢ ἐντεῦθεν. περὶ μὲν οὖν ὅλου τοῦ πρήγματος ἀρκεῖ μοι ταῦτα· μετὰ δὲ ταῦτα πρὸς αὐτὰ τὰ ἔργα τῷ αὐτῷ λόγῳ πορευθεὶς ἐπιδείξω τὰ νοσήματα τούτου ἔκγονα πάντα ἐόντα.

> Now I have said that all animals participate largely in air. So after this I must say that it is likely that maladies occur from this source and from no other. On the subject as a whole I have said sufficient; after this I will by the same reasoning proceed to facts and show that diseases are all the offspring of air.

> *(On Breaths*, 5.1–2)

As well as indicating what has been said and what will be said – structuring the discussion and emphasising the points being made – the author empha-sises the sufficiency of what has been said, and in this way implies mastery of the subject. As in *On the Nature of Human Beings*, signposting is also used to build suspense.

The use of a lively, simple style may be engaging for a non-expert and the attention to phonic features such as use of rhythm shows the influence of oral and musical communication methods. The phrase 'μετὰ δὲ ταῦτα πρὸς αὐτὰ τὰ ἔργα τῷ αὐτῷ λόγῳ πορευθεὶς ἐπιδείξω τὰ νοσήματα τούτου ἔκγονα πάντα ἐόντα', for instance, includes a high proportion of short-syllabled words, from which a hint of a pattern emerges with strings of two-syllable words followed by single-syllable words. The shortness of the words and the frequency of 'α' help to communicate a sense of rapidity.

It certainly seems highly plausible that these features could have been exploited in a performance context, and the subject matter and tone suggests a lay audience, perhaps a large crowd. Nevertheless, this does not preclude the possibility of the treatise being read by individuals and for multiple uses of individual treatises; it does, however, indicate influence of and reference to earlier prose works more thoroughly embedded within the tradition of sound patterning to convey meaning.

We have seen in the discussion above, then, that while there are references to display and demonstration and features of oral style which are broadly similar in the Hippocratic oratorical treatises, close examination of verbal references to display and demonstration and consideration of the presence of signposting as a feature of oral style do not yield any definitive insights into the nature of Hippocratic oratory, though we do gain glimpses and suggestive hints as to possible performance context. As noted at the beginning of this chapter, an understanding of the genre of epideictic based solely on Aristotle's definition in the *Rhetoric* misses the complex earlier history of expository prose; analysis in this chapter of the use of terms indicating 'display' and 'demonstrate' and the use of signposting in the selected Hippocratic treatises indicates that each author is working to define for himself the explanatory and expressive framework in which his case is being made.

The individuality of each text and each author impresses itself upon us, with, in many cases, differences in the references to display and demonstration and in the use of signposting showing that each author approaches the question of how to communicate with an audience rather differently; this in turn implies a range of performance contexts and persuasive aims and the absence of a clearly defined genre or standard of expository prose.

As already noted above, in the following chapters I go on to explore further features which have been attributed to oral style by Gagarin, namely use of sound and antithetical constructions. In Chapter 4, I focus on phonic features in *On Breaths* and closely related models for these in the extant literature which precedes the composition of this treatise.

Notes

1 See for example Demont (1993) and Thomas (2003); see also Carey (2007).

2 Loraux goes on to explain the limitation of using Aristotle as a basis for analysis of Greek prose, with reference to her subject of study: 'It is not in Aristotle's inevitably classificatory thought, but in a study of the funeral oration itself, regarded as a fixed form and as a genre made up of *topoi*, that we must look for an answer to the question of its status' (2006 [1986]: 284).

3 'd'un côté, l'exposé oral didactique ou "cours"; de l'autre, l'exposé oral épidictique ou "discours"'.

4 Aristotle, *Rhetoric* 1409a24–37: 'τὴν δὲ λέξιν ἀνάγκη εἶναι ἢ εἰρομένην καὶ τῷ συνδέσμῳ μίαν, ὥσπερ αἱ ἐν τοῖς διθυράμβοις ἀναβολαί, ἢ κατεστραμμένην καὶ ὁμοίαν ταῖς τῶν ἀρχαίων ποιητῶν ἀντιστρόφοις. ἡ μὲν οὖν εἰρομένη λέξις ἡ ἀρχαία ἐστίν "Ἡροδότου Θουρίου ἥδ᾽ ἱστορίης ἀπόδειξις" (ταύτῃ γὰρ πρότερον μὲν ἅπαντες, νῦν δὲ οὐ πολλοὶ χρῶνται): λέγω δὲ εἰρομένην ἢ οὐδὲν ἔχει τέλος καθ᾽ αὑτήν, ἂν μὴ τὸ πρᾶγμα τὸ λεγόμενον τελειωθῇ. ἔστι δὲ ἀηδὴς διὰ τὸ ἄπειρον: τὸ γὰρ τέλος πάντες βούλονται καθορᾶν: διόπερ ἐπὶ τοῖς καμπτῆρσιν ἐκπνέουσι καὶ ἐκλύονται: προορῶντες γὰρ τὸ πέρας οὐ κάμνουσι πρότερον. ἡ μὲν οὖν εἰρομένη τῆς λέξεώς ἐστιν ἥδε, κατεστραμμένη δὲ ἡ ἐν περιόδοις: λέγω δὲ περίοδον λέξιν ἔχουσαν ἀρχὴν καὶ τελευτὴν αὐτὴν καθ᾽ αὑτὴν καὶ μέγεθος εὐσύνοπτον.'

'The style must be either continuous and united by connecting particles, like the dithyrambic preludes, or periodic, like the antistrophes of the ancient poets. The continuous style is the ancient one; for example, "This is the exposition of the investigation of Herodotus of Thurii." It was formerly used by all, but now is used only by a few. By a continuous style I mean that which has no end in itself and only stops when the sense is complete. It is unpleasant, because it is endless, for all wish to have the end in sight. That explains why runners, just when they have reached the goal, lose their breath and strength, whereas before, when the end is in sight, they show no signs of fatigue. Such is the continuous style. The other style consists of periods, and by period I mean a sentence that has a beginning and end in itself and a magnitude that can be easily grasped' (Freese 1926).

5 The 'peroration' is essentially a conclusion or epilogue to a work; see Lausberg (1998: §§431–442).

6 Gagarin, in his chapter on oratory and rhetoric before the Sophists notes that 'there is no evidence [before the fourth century BCE] to suggest the systematic study or analysis of the practice of public speaking beyond the simple observation of individuals' manners of speaking. Rhetoric in the fourth-century sense is still lacking' (2006: 30). See also Mann's comments on *epideixis* in relation to *On the Art* (2012: 17–18): he argues that in this treatise we find a pre-Aristotelian notion of *epideixis*.

7 He refers to Isocrates' *Helen*, Gorgias' *Olympic Discourse* and Isocrates *Panegyricus* in discussing *prooimia* of epideictic speeches (3. 14, 1–2).

8 The German title is 'Die Epideixis über die Techne im V. und IV. Jh.'.

9 'Gegenüber, *Epideixis*' führt der Begriff '*Genos epideiktikon*' zwei Besonderheiten ein. Erstens ist es natürlich nur eine Art Redekunst. Zweistens unterscheidet sich meistens der Redner von dem Mann, dessen Trefflichkeit gelobt wird'.

10 G. Kennedy, in his edition of Aristotle's *Rhetoric* notes: 'Epideictic discourse, in particular, needs to be looked at in a variety of ways not recognised by Aristotle. He thought of it as the rhetoric of praise or blame, as in a funeral oration or a denunciation of someone, and failed to formulate its role in the instilling, preservation, or enhancement of cultural values, even though this was a major function,

as seen in Pericles' famous funeral oration or the epideictic speeches of Isocrates. His apparent lack of interest in the moral value of epideictic rhetoric is perhaps influenced by scorn for Isocrates, but it is also analogous to his feelings about poetry' (1991: 22).

11 cf. Dodds' comments on Plato *Gorgias*, 447 A 5 (1959: 189).

12 *De articulis* XXXV, IV 158–160 in Littré, 1973–1989 [1839–1861] (II 155 Kühle-wein)

13 'In solchen Vorträgen, wie etwa auch in *De morb. sac.* und *De nat. hom.*, bedeutet der Gebrauch dieser Verben nur, daß der Fachmann seine Fähigkeiten und seine Theorien zugleich vorweisen und beweisen möchte.'

14 See above, pp. 5-7 (Chapter 1) and pp. 59–62.

15 See Liddell and Scott (1996).

16 ἐπίδειξις, ἡ: I. ostentatio *De Arte* 6,32,4; *Vict* I 6,496,8; *Praec* 9,266,14; II. demonstratio (pl.) *De Arte* 6,26,9. ἐπιδεικνύμι: I. exhibeo *Prog* 2,134,1; *demonstro* VM 1,572,15.16; *Art* 4,158,13; *Flat* 6,96,18 and 114,15,16; *Vict* I 6,468,5; *Decent* 9,242,5; *VM* 1,620,10; demonstratio *De Arte* 6,26,10 (Kühn et al. 1986). References to Hippocratic treatises are listed as they appear in the *Index Hippocraticus*, to the Littré edition of the Hippocratic Collection.

17 These are, in the order in which they are discussed in this chapter: *On the Sacred Disease*, 1.3; *On Breaths*, 1.5; 15.1; 15.2; *On the Sacred Disease*, 1.13; *On the Art*, 3.1–3; 2. 2; *On the Nature of Human Beings*, 2.4–5; *On Ancient Medicine* 2.2; *On the Art,* 13.1; *On Ancient Medicine* 19.7–20.1; *On the Art*, 10.4. See also *On the Nature of Human Beings* 5.3–4; *On the Art* 1.1 and *Airs, Waters, Places*, 12, 1–2.

18 This use of ἀποδείκνυμι does seem to offer some support for Bakker's argument that the term is used to denote a response to a specific situation, that it deals in differentiation (in this case the need is to distinguish between religious and non-religious territory) and that what is shown is always changed in the act and may not even have existed before in (2002: 20–28).

19 Thomas notes with reference to this use of the term that 'it is the ἀπόδειξις of a particular theory, but it seems, like the English "display" and ἐπιδείξις, to be shading off into a "demonstration piece"' (2003: 252).

20 This use of ἀπόδειξις here does accord with the idea put forward by Bakker that the term indicates 'an act that is performed in response to a specific situation' (2002: 21) – the specific situation being the response to critics of medicine. However, *On Breaths* uses 'ἐπίδειξις' to the same purpose.

21 This sense of statement and supporting explanation indicated by the terms φημί and ἀποδείκνυμι respectively occurs again later in the same treatise: 'συγγέγονε δὲ ταῦτα τὰ εἰρημένα· πῶς γὰρ οὐ ξυγγέγονε; πρῶτον μὲν φανερός ἐστιν ὤνθρωπος ἔχων ἐν ἑωυτῷ ταῦτα πάντα αἴδια ἕως ἂν ζῆ, ἔπειτα δὲ γέγονεν ἐξ ἀνθρώπου ταῦτα πάντα ἔχοντος, τέθραπταί τε ἐν ἀνθρώπῳ ταῦτα πάντα ἔχοντι, ὅσα ἐγὼ φημί τε καὶ ἀποδείκνυμι.' 'The named elements are congenital: for how could they not be? For firstly it is obvious that a human being has all these elements inside perpetually as long as he or she is alive; secondly, human beings are born and nourished inside other human beings who have all these elements as well, that is those elements that I now state and demonstrate' (5, 3–4).

22 See e.g. Connors (1986), Havelock (1986: 46–47) for further work on the orality of oratory; see also Thomas (1992).

23 Gagarin notes that 'Before the second half of the fifth century oratory was entirely oral – composed and performed ex tempore, and not preserved except for the occasional memorable phrase . . . or the fictional versions of poets and historians.

The earliest speeches to be written were composed by sophists and logographers' (1998: 164).

24 On the term 'parallelism': '[it] has been coined in relatively recent times, and it does not belong to the traditional terminology of rhetoric. It usually designates a group of discursive phenomena, both of a formal and semantic nature, known since ancient times under the Greek terms *parison* and *parisōsis*' Mayoral and Ballesteros (2001; 552–553). Lausberg describes *parison* and *parisōsis* as follows: 'Isocolon, or parison, or parisosis consists in the coordinated juxtaposition of two or more colons or commas, whereby generally speaking the colons (or commas) each manifest the same sentence sequence. The colons themselves can be syntactically complete main or subordinate clauses or (also in the case of commas) consist of in each case at least two-element sentence parts, which are integrated into the sentence as a "parenthesis" by means of a further sentence part' (1998: 320).

References

Bakker, E. J. (2002), 'The Making of History: Herodotus' Historiês Apodexis' in Bakker, E. J., de Jong, I, J, F, and van Wees, H. (eds.), *Brill's Companion to Herodotus*. Leiden: Brill. 3–32.

Carey, C. (2007), 'Epideictic Oratory' in Worthington, I. (ed.), *A Companion to Greek Rhetoric*. Oxford: Blackwell. 236–252.

Connors, R. J. (1986), 'Greek Rhetoric and the Transition from Orality.' *Philosophy & Rhetoric*. Penn State University Press. 19(1): 38–65.

Dean-Jones, L. (2003), 'Literacy and the Charlatan in Ancient Greek Medicine' in Yunis, H. (ed.), *Written Texts and the Rise of Literate Culture*. Cambridge: Cambridge University Press. 97–121.

Demont, P. (1993), 'Die Epideixis über die Techne im V. und IV. Jh.' in Kullmann, W. and Althoff, J. (eds.), *Vermittlung und Tradieren von Wissen in der griechischen Kultur*. Tübingen: G. Narr. 181–209.

Dodds, E. R. (1959), *Plato. Gorgias*. A Revised Text with Introduction and Commentary. Oxford: Clarendon Press.

Freese, J. H. (trans.) (1926), *Aristotle. Rhetoric*. London: W. Heinemann; New York: G. P. Putnam's Sons.

Gagarin, M. (2006), 'Background and Origins: Oratory and Rhetoric before the Sophists' in Worthington, I. (ed.), *A Companion to Greek Rhetoric*. Malden, MA; Oxford: Blackwell Publications. 27–36.

Gagarin, M. (1998), 'The Orality of Greek Oratory' in Mackay, E. A. (ed.), *Signs of Orality: The Oral Tradition and Its Influence in the Greek and Roman World*. Leiden: Brill. 163–180.

Gagarin, M. (ed.) (1997), *Antiphon: The Speeches*. Cambridge: Cambridge University Press.

Havelock, E. A. (1986), *The Muse Learns to Write: Reflections on Orality and Literacy from Antiquity to the Present*. New Haven, CT: Yale University Press.

Jouanna, J. (ed. and trans.) (2003), *Hippocrate. Tome II, 3e partie. La maladie sacrée*. Paris: Les Belles Lettres.

Jouanna, J. (ed. and trans.) (1988), *Hippocrate. Tome V, 1re partie. Des vents; De l'art*. Paris: Les Belles Lettres.

Jouanna, J. (1984), 'Rhétorique et médecine dans la collection Hippocratique: contribution à l'histoire de la rhétorique au Ve siècle.' *Revue des Études greques* 97. Paris: Société d'Edition 'Les Belles Lettres'. 26–44.

Kennedy, G. A. (trans.) (1991), *Aristotle. On Rhetoric: A Theory of Civic Discourse*. New York; Oxford: Oxford University Press.

Lausberg, H. (1998), *Handbook of Literary Rhetoric: A Foundation for Literary Study*; translated by M. T. Bliss, A. Jansen, D. E. Orton; edited by D. E. Orton and R. D. Anderson. Leiden; Boston, MA: Brill.

Liddell, H. G. and Scott, R. (eds.) (1996), *A Greek–English Lexicon*. Oxford: Clarendon Press.

Littré, É. (ed. and trans.) (1973–1989 [1839–1861]), *Œuvres complètes d'Hippocrate*. Amsterdam: Adolf M. Hakkert. Reprint of Paris : J. B. Baillière, 1839–1861.

Loraux, N. (2006 [1986]), *The Invention of Athens: The Funeral Oration in the Classical City*; translated from the French by A. Sheridan. New York: Zone Books; Cambridge, MA: distributed by the MIT Press.

Mann, J. E. (2012), *Hippocrates, On the Art of Medicine*. Leiden; Boston, MA: Brill.

Mayoral, J. A., and Ballesteros, A. (2001), 'Parellelism' in Sloane, T. L. (ed.), *Encyclopedia of Rhetoric*. Oxford: Oxford University Press.

Thomas, R. (2003), 'Prose Performance Texts: *Epideixis* and Written Publication in the Late Fifth and Early Fourth Centuries' in Yunis, H. (ed.), *Written Texts and the Rise of Literate Culture in Ancient Greece*. Cambridge: Cambridge University Press. 162–188.

Thomas, R. (2000), *Herodotus in Context: Ethnography, Science and the Art of Persuasion*. Cambridge: Cambridge University Press.

Thomas, R. (1992), *Literacy and Orality in Ancient Greece*. Cambridge: Cambridge University Press.

4 Gorgias, Heraclitus and the persuasive functions of sound in *On Breaths*

This chapter will explore persuasive patterns and the relationship between form and content in Gorgias' *Encomium of Helen*, a key example of Sophistic prose, and extant fragments of Heraclitus' writing in light of the analysis of *On Breaths*, which, as will become clear in the chapter, has the strongest connection with these examples of Sophistic and pre-Socratic prose of the five Hippocratic treatises focused on in this book.

We saw, in Chapter 2, how Hippocratic expository prose mixes persuasive patterning and elements of argument from evidence to develop a new kind of medical *logos* in which writers put forward a case through meanings built up associatively and implicitly, as well as through the linear logic of argument. We also saw, in Chapter 3, how there is evidence in the five selected Hippocratic treatises of each author seeking to establish their own manner of communicating with an audience and suggestions as to a range of performance contexts.

In this chapter, I focus on *On Breaths* as a case study, and analyse closely the use of sound patterning in expository prose. As well as exploring the presence of sonic resonances in the treatise, I examine in further detail the relationship between this treatise and that of the work of earlier models of prose writing, arguing that *On Breaths* looks back to the earlier Ionian work of Heraclitus for useful expressive resources, and also moves in some sort of parallel with the probably nearly contemporary work of Gorgias. Establishing this larger pattern should help us to gain a better understanding of the expressive resources deployed in Heraclitus' and Gorgias' expository prose, as well as in that of the Hippocratic treatise *On Breaths*, and by implication provide some further insight into the relationship between these authors' work.

Let us firstly consider briefly Jouanna's comments on the relationship between Gorgias' *Encomium of Helen* and *On Breaths*. Jouanna states in his article on rhetoric and the Hippocratic Collection that there is a significant relationship between the treatises *On Breaths*, *On the Art* and *Encomium of Helen* in that they are all rare examples of epideictic oratory and share many persuasive characteristics (Jouanna 1984: 38). In both his article on rhetoric and the Hippocratic Collection and his edition of *On Breaths*, he notes the particularly close proximity of *Encomium of Helen* and *On Breaths*: 'no work, in the preserved literature, is as close to *Encomium of Helen* as the treatise *On Breaths*' (Jouanna 1988: 11; cf. Jouanna 1984: 38 f.).[1]

As noted in the previous chapter, Jouanna states overall that *On the Art*, *On Breaths* and *Encomium of Helen* all correspond to a definition of epide-ictic discourse according to Aristotle (Jouanna 1984: 36–38). He notes that various aspects of the composition of *On Breaths* are similar to *Encomium of Helen*: he points out, for instance, that *On the Art* and *On Breaths* are the only treatises in the collection to have a developed preamble and conclusion, like *Encomium of Helen* (Jouanna 1988: 13). Jouanna also points to the use of verbs in the first person and of rhetorical questions; the didactic character of the writing; the similarity of transitions between sections; the classification and ordering of arguments and the way demonstrations are introduced as signs of the close relationship between the two treatises (Jouanna 1988: 13–17).

He notes that the concise parallel or antithetical phrasing found in *On Breaths* and *Encomium of Helen* indicates a very close relationship between these two texts, closer than the one between *On the Art* and *Encomium of Helen*, stating that 'The main characteristic of periodic style is the use of antithesis that places two clauses of a phrase of the same length (parisosis) ending in the same sounds (paromoiosis) in opposition' (Jouanna 1984: 37).[2] He also notes that both *On Breaths* and *Encomium of Helen* deal with praise and blame (*On Breaths* is a eulogy to the power of air; *Encomium of Helen* to the power of *logos*) (Jouanna 1984: 38–40; cf. Jouanna 1988: 13).

Jouanna goes on to note the presence and use of play on sound in *On Breaths* and *Encomium of Helen*. Both texts are shown to employ the repeated use of rhetorical questions, the use of imagined objections from the audience, an attempt at clarity, the same manner of announcements of the subject of their discourse and similar transitions between sections of the text (Jouanna 1988: 13–16). Jouanna also notes here that the authors divide up points within their arguments in the same way, show a similar subdivision of key notions into categories, introduce evidence in the same way and also end their treatises in a similar fashion (Jouanna 1988: 16–17).

Jouanna gives a long list of examples of comparisons and metaphors in *On Breaths* and *Encomium of Helen* that he states contribute to their identi-fication with 'poetic prose' of which Aristotle gives Gorgias as an example (Jouanna 1988: 18–19).[3] He claims that 'many of these images have their ori-gin in technical Ionic prose that seems naturally similar and whose expression, which is called poetic, may derive less from imitation of poetry (epic, lyric or tragic) than from the riches of the common Ionian treasury of prose and poetry' (Jouanna 1988: 19).[4]

Jouanna goes on to list instances of the presence of *paromoion* (alliteration) and *parison* (even balance between the members of a sentence) and in partic-ular notes the many examples of doubling found in both treatises.[5] Examples of play on the sound of words found in the succession and accumulation of words which have an identical or analogous sound are listed next (Jouanna 1988: 22–23). Jouanna remarks in passing that

> the repetition of the same term to interlink phrases and to mark the stages of an argument and of a physiological process, as when 14.2 (p.122, line 1) ψυχθέντι δὲ τῷ αἵματι ['once the blood is cooled'] repeats τὸ αἷμα ψύχεται ['the blood cools'], is a characteristic of Ionian prose that has not undergone Sophistic influence.
>
> (Jouanna 1988: 23–24)[6]

Finally, he notes the presence of *parechema* (words which have the same sound but are not formed on the same root) and alliteration in the treatise, as well as two examples of prose meter found in *On Breaths* (Jouanna 1988: 24).[7]

As discussed in the first and third chapters of this study, it is anachronistic to use Aristotle's definition of epideictic discourse to judge the correspondence of these texts; more importantly for this chapter, absent from Jouanna's discussion is a sense of the interplay between form and content that exists in these texts and is arguably another aspect of the connection between them. The following comments seek to identify some of the main features of interplay between form and content in *Encomium of Helen* and *On Breaths* by way of complement to Jounna's analysis of the connection between the two texts and to extend our understanding of the relationship of *On Breaths* with contemporary writing.

(a) Gorgias' Encomium of Helen

> Κόσμος πόλει μὲν εὐανδρία, σώματι δὲ κάλλος, ψύχῃι δὲ σοφία, πράγματι δὲ ἀρετή, λόγωι δὲ ἀλήθεια· τὰ δὲ ἐναντία τούτων ἀκοσμία. ἄνδρα δὲ καὶ γυναῖκα καὶ λόγον καὶ ἔργον καὶ πόλιν καὶ πρᾶγμα χρὴ τὸ μὲν ἄξιον ἐπαίνου ἐπαίνωι τιμᾶν, τῶι δὲ ἀναξίωι μῶμον ἐπιτιθέναι· ἴσε γὰρ ἁμαρτία καὶ ἀμαθία μέμφεσθαί τε τὰ ἐπαινετὰ καὶ ἐπαινεῖν τὰ μωμητά.

> The order of a city lies in the quality of its men, of a body in beauty, of a mind in wisdom, of an object in excellence, of a speech in truth. The opposites of these qualities constitute disorderliness. If a man, a woman, a speech, a deed, a city, and an object deserve praise one should honour them with praise, but if they do not one should apply blame. For it is an equal failure and ignorance to blame things which are to be praised and to approve things which are to be censured.
>
> (*Encomium of Helen*, 1 in Waterfield 2009 [2000]: 228)

In this, the opening of *Encomium of Helen*, we find a balanced and repetitive sentence structure which embodies orderliness; the topic discussed – orderliness – is in this way reflected and expressed in the form of the phrasing used. We also find the list structure and the use of oppositions supporting the idea of a neat and orderly categorisation. The term 'ἐναντία' 'opposites' is used in the above extract to make a generalisation about order in able-bodied men, bodies, the soul and affairs. The term emphasises the presence of opposition in the word order of the sentence and treats these verbal oppositions as if they were themselves evidence which can be used to construct a generalisation. Gorgias is saying that, because he can find a number of examples of opposition which he can convey through his writing, it is 'valid' to make a generalisation about the nature of this opposition.

We find a similar technique used in *On Breaths* where oppositions are first verbalised – e.g. 'Τί οὖν λιμοῦ φάρμακον; Ὅ παύει λιμόν' (1.4) – and then a generalisation is made on the basis of this verbalisation, for example: 'τὰ ἐναντία τῶν ἐναντίων ἐστὶν ἰήματα' 'opposites are the remedy for opposites' (1.5), and 'Εἰ γάρ τις εἰδείη τὴν αἰτίην τοῦ νοσήματος, οἷός τ'ἂν εἴη τὰ συμφέροντα προσφέρειν τῷ σώματι ἐκ τῶν ἐναντίων ἐπιστάμενος τῷ νοσήματι' 'If one knows the cause of the disease, one would be able to administer to the body whatever is useful, bring opposites to oppose the disease.' (1.4). The oppositions that are described serve as the foundation for the generalisation that then goes on to be made.

Jouanna does not comment on the use of the term 'ἐναντία' in the phrases cited above, though he does note that the phrase from *On Breaths* 'τὰ ἐναντία τῶν ἐναντίων ἐστὶν ἰήματα' 'opposites are the remedy for opposites' (1.5) is an example of polyptoton (words derived from the same stem being repeated) which is common in *Encomium of Helen* (Jouanna 1988: 22). Without linking the form with the content here, we miss the method that these authors are using both to establish evidence and to argue their case.

Furthermore, the structure of the oppositions verbalised in *On Breaths* – for example, the 'a-b, b-a' structure of the phrase: 'πόνον δὲ ἀπονίη, ἀπονίην δὲ πόνος' 'exercise [is cured by] rest, rest by exercise' (1.4) – implies a neat balance which endows the generalisation, when it is made, with a sense of balance, neatness and order; we find the same strategy in the opening of Gorgias' *Encomium of Helen*. The use of alpha privative is also characteristic in both examples in the context of black and white, balanced oppositions. We find, for instance 'τὰ δὲ ἐναντία τούτων ἀκοσμία' 'The opposites of these things are disorderliness' in the passage above from *Encomium of Helen* that recalls the use of alpha privative in the line from *On Breaths* quoted immediately above.

We find further examples in *Encomium of Helen* that echo persuasive strategies that I have identified in *On Breaths*. We have seen that Gorgias presents black and white oppositions; he also characterises the opinion of the poets about Helen as homogenous using the adjectives 'ὁμόφωνος' 'in accordance' and 'ὁμόψυχος' 'unanimous' in Section 2. We also find in this section a sense of a straightforward conflict between truth and falsehood – another black and white opposition:

> ἐγὼ δὲ βούλομαι λογισμόν τινα τῶι λόγωι δοὺς τὴν μὲν κακῶς ἀκούούσαν παῦσαι τῆς αἰτίας, τοὺς δὲ μεμφομένους ψευδομένους ἐπιδείξας καὶ δείξας τἀληθὲς [ἢ] παῦσαι τῆς ἀμαθίας.

> I would like, by means of the logic with which I shall inform my speech, to free both the slandered woman from the charges against her and her detractors from their ignorance, by demonstrating the falsity of their views and by revealing the truth.
>
>   (*Encomium of Helen*, 2 in Waterfield 2009 [2000]: 228)

In *Encomium of Helen*, then, there is a conflict between opposites that is played out at the conceptual as well as the linguistic level, just as in *On Breaths* opposition has a role to play at the conceptual level of how medicine works which is reflected in the play on language.

Another aspect of the closeness of the kinship between *Encomium of Helen* and *On Breaths* is word play. Although there is a lot of play on sound and word order in Gorgias' *Encomium of Helen*, as Jouanna has pointed out, this is confined in most examples to sonorous pairs and accumulations of words that do not have a direct bearing on the play between form and content in this treatise.

As well as the sonorous pairs and the accumulations of words, there are also various examples in *On Breaths* of expressions that involve repetition of pairs of near synonyms. Jouanna notes many of these in his discussion, cited above; two representative examples are as follows (1988: 20–24). We find 'παχύνεται καὶ πυκνοῦνται' 'thickens and condenses' when the author is describing the way that steam turns to water under the lid of a saucepan of boiling water as an analogy for the occurrence of perspiration (8.6). The phrase 'πλησθεῖσαι δὲ καὶ πρησθεῖσαι' 'full and swollen' is used to describe the state of vessels when headaches occur during fevers (8.7). These pairs of words, which tend to echo one another in sound, seem to provide an extra level of precision to the vocabulary which is not at this stage very technical: nuances of meaning can be produced by using a pair of words as opposed to just one word. The connection in sound reflects and so helps to naturalise, or knit together, their connection in terms of meaning, but they do not connect with the argument of the treatise directly in the way that we have seen with the use of oppositions above.

It is important to bear in mind that as well as similarities between the two treatises, there are also striking differences. In *Encomium of Helen*, for instance, the persuasive power of language itself is praised:

λόγος δυνάστης μέγας ἐστίν, ὃς σμικροτάτωι σώματι καὶ ἀφανεστάτωι θειότατα ἔργα ἀποτελεῖ· δύναται γὰρ καὶ φόβον παῦσαι καὶ λύπην ἀφελεῖν καὶ χαρὰν ἐνεργάσασθαι καὶ ἔλεον ἐπαυξῆσαι. ταῦτα δὲ ὡς οὕτως ἔχει δείξω·

The spoken word is a mighty lord, and for all that it is insubstantial and imperceptible it has superhuman effects. It can put an end to fear, do away with distress, generate happiness, and increase pity. I will now prove that this is so.

(*Encomium of Helen*, 8 in Waterfield 2009 [2000]: 229)

As Jouanna notes, this reminds us of the praise of the power of air in *On Breaths* – 'Οὗτος δὲ μέγιστος ἐν τοῖσι πᾶσι τῶν πάντων δυνάστης ἐστίν.' 'It is a very powerful master that reigns in every way over everything.' (3.2) (Jouanna 1988: 13). Furthermore, to add to the sense of there being a connection between *Encomium of Helen* and *On Breaths* is the notion of praising air or speech: both texts describe their object of praise as invisible. In the above quotations, speech is portrayed as an invisible and divine being and in *On Breaths* air is depicted as 'ὄψει ἀφανής, τῷ δὲ λογισμῷ φανερός' 'invisible to the eye but visible to reason' (3.3).

Despite the clear parallels here, the fact that Gorgias praises speech and the author of *On Breaths* praises air suggests that *Encomium of Helen* has a different relationship with language from *On Breaths*. While *On Breaths* may be heavily influenced by Sophistic techniques, this is not to say that it does not also have a serious message to convey about the nature of medicine; Gorgias' *Encomium of Helen*, by contrast, is a mock defence because it treats a mythological figure.

(b) Repetition of sounds and phrases in On Breaths

We find some uses of phonetic repetition in *On Breaths* that have no obvious parallels in *Encomium of Helen*. For example:

Ὁ δὲ τοῦτ' ἄριστα ποιέων ἄριστος ἰητρός, ὁ δὲ τούτου πλεῖστον ἀπολειφθεὶς πλεῖστον ἀπελείφθη τῆς τέχνης.

Whoever carries this out best is the best physician, whoever is furthest from it is furthest from the art.

(*On Breaths*, 1.5)

Here, the phrase 'πλεῖστον ἀπολειφθείς' 'furthest from it [with a passive participle]' is almost exactly repeated in the phrase 'πλεῖστον ἀπελείφθη' 'furthest from it [with the verb in the passive voice]'. The repetition is memorable and emphasises the point being made that the best physician manages most skilfully the addition of what is lacking and the removal of what is in excess, which this author defines as the essence of the medical art.

Another example of fairly straightforward repetition of sounds is the following example from the author's account of epidemic fever:

> Ὁ μὲν πολύκοινος πυρετὸς διὰ τοῦτο τοιοῦτός ἐστιν, ὅτι τὸ πνεῦμα τωὐτὸ πάντες ἕλκουσιν· ὁμοίου δὲ ὁμοίως τοῦ πνεύματος τῷ σώματι μιχθέντος, ὅμοιοι καὶ οἱ πυρετοὶ γίνονται.

> Common fever is common to all because the air which all breathe in is the same: when air which is similar mixes in a similar fashion with the body, similar fevers arise.
>
> (*On Breaths*, 6.2)

Here the word 'ὁμοίος' is used firstly as an adjective, then as an adverb, then again as an adjective in slightly different contexts (the types of air; the manner of mixing and the types of fever) building up the notion of 'sameness'. The term 'ὁμοίος' and its variants are also reinforced with the nearly synonymous – but not 'homonymous' (i.e. pronounced the same) – words 'πολύκοινος' 'common' and 'τωὐτὸ' 'the same'. The repetition of different words – some of which also sound similar – with the same or nearly the same meaning helps to emphasise the idea that this fever is the same for all.[8]

There are some examples of repetition of words to mark the stages in a process, as in the following:

> Ὁπόταν γυμνασθὲν ὑπὸ τῶν πόνων τὸ σῶμα θερμανθῇ, θερμαίνεται καὶ τὸ αἷμα· τὸ δὲ αἷμα διαθερμανθὲν ἐξεθέρμηνε τὰς φύσας· αὗται δὲ διαθερμανθεῖσαι διαλύονται καὶ διαλύουσιν τὴν σύστασιν τοῦ αἵματος

> Whenever after exercising, the body is heated up from exertion, the blood is also heated up; the blood once it is well heated heats the air; the air, once it is well heated is dispersed and disperses the accumulation of blood
>
> (*On Breaths*, 14.7)

The repetition of the term 'θερμαίνω' in various different forms emphasises the different stages in the process and underlines the coherence of these developments as part of a single process; the repetition of different forms of the verb in different tenses marking the different stages in the process, and the sound of the main stem of the word offering a sense of continuity.

The linking repetitions which emphasise and embody the chain of cause and effect which the author is describing also extends to the triple use of the schema subordinate aorist followed by main verb: Ὁπόταν . . . θερμανθῇ, θερμαίνεται . . . διαθερμανθὲν ἐξεθέρμηνε . . . διαθερμανθεῖσαι διαλύονται’ ‘Whenever . . . [it] is heated up, [the blood] is heated up . . . [the blood] well heated heats . . . [the air] well heated disperses’. Furthermore, we find the insistent repetition of ‘δια-’ (which moreover as a prefix in compounds can indicate ‘in succession’ (as in ‘διαδέχομαι’ ‘to receive from another’, ‘to succeed’) as well as ‘thoroughly’ (which is the surface meaning here). Finally, in the sequence ‘διαλύονται καὶ διαλύουσιν’ ‘is dispersed and disperses’ the shift from passive to active form of the same verb emphasises the closeness of the connection being described here between the dispersal of air and the dispersal of blood.

If we consider another author whose work is notorious for playing on the relationship between form and content and who could have been an influence on *On Breaths*, we find further insight into the kinds of techniques *On Breaths* is employing, rather than making a comparison with *Encomium of Helen* alone. It is this more elaborate sense of the relationship between form and content that interests me here. Let us consider next, then, the writing of Heraclitus.

(c) On Breaths *and the writing of Heraclitus*

Heraclitus is one of the earliest writers of prose of whose work evidence is extant: he is renowned for his manipulation of language to express subtle, complex and often deliberately enigmatic meaning.[9] Although we cannot be sure of the relationship between Heraclitus’ writing and that of the Hippocratics and the evidence we have for Heraclitus’ work cannot be securely dated, similarities in the writing of Heraclitus can be discerned in *On Breaths* and *On the Sacred Disease* as well as on many other contemporary authors: the Hippocratic treatises *Nutriment* and *Regimen I*, for instance, clearly show reflections of the style found in Heraclitus’ writing.[10] Gorgias is also thought to have been influenced by the Heraclitean notion of ‘λόγος’ (see below).[11] There need not necessarily be a direct influence, nor need the evidence of Heraclitus’ writing be provably authentic for this comparison to be fruitful because it can in any case shed further light on the persuasive techniques in play in the Hippocratic treatises.

Kahn’s useful analysis of three main areas of language use in Heraclitus covers punning, syntactic play and resonance; he describes these as features of language use related to aspects of Heraclitus’ philosophical theories.[12] Let us here, by way of introduction, identify some characteristic illustrations of Heraclitus' use of language, and two examples showing the use of language in *On Breaths* and *On the Sacred Disease* that are reminiscent of his work in general. We will then examine specifically the use of sound in *On Breaths* and examples from this treatise where the author appears to be making direct reference to Heraclitus.

The extant opening of Heraclitus' book expresses the notion, implicitly prevalent throughout his writing, that there is a parallelism between the structure of the account of the world which he gives and the nature of the world itself. He writes 'τοῦ δὲ λόγου τοῦδ᾽ ἐόντος ἀεὶ' 'This account holds forever' and 'γινομένων γὰρ πάντων κατὰ τὸν λόγον τόνδε' 'all things come to pass in accordance with this account'.[13] The meaning of the word 'λόγος' can be read as ambiguous here: it may refer both to the underlying structure or reason that Heraclitus understands is omnipresent in the universe and to the author's own account of this structure or reason, for Heraclitus thinks that 'The whole world is intelligent and alive, and speaks to the wise man subtly, communicating its inner nature and enabling him to model himself on it' (Waterfield 2009: 32).

This appears to be an example of Heraclitus punning on the word 'λόγος' (i.e. using the word to mean more than one thing) and using this pun to pinpoint the parallel between the written account and the nature of the world that is at the heart of the author's philosophical outlook. Although there is no direct parallel for such a notion in *On Breaths*, we have seen above how both Gorgias and the author of *On Breaths* use verbalised oppositions as 'evidence' on which to make a generalisation.

One of the more complexly structured of Heraclitus' fragments is an illustration of the author manipulating syntax in order to make a point about the nature of life and death and about epistemology. The use of language in this fragment is much more like the use of language we find in the Hippocratic authors.

> ἀθάνατοι θνητοί, θνητοὶ ἀθάνατοι, ζῶντες τὸν ἐκείνων θάνατον, τὸν δὲ ἐκείνων βίον τεθνεῶτες.

> Immortal mortals, mortal immortals, living the death of these, dying the life of those.[14]

This sentence expresses the relationship, as understood by Heraclitus, between life and death and mortal and immortal by employing an 'a-b, b-a' pattern twice in the arrangement of the words; the simple repetition of the words in the first half of the sentence also makes a neat phonetic effect that emphasises the chiasmus. Heraclitus puts the opposite terms alongside one another in order to suggest that their opposition may be undermined (there is very little space between the words on the page just as there is very little distance between their conceptual meaning) and that there is some level of equivalence between them. The opposition is enigmatic: by implying that the opposite terms may be equivalent, the author aims to unsettle the reader's or listener's understanding of these terms (which would normally be considered contrasting pairs of opposites) and to question the fundamental meaning of the terms and so to embark upon philosophical enquiry.[15]

The difficulty of interpreting Heraclitus' meaning here – 'immortals are mortals, mortals immortal' seems to be a paradox – reflects the difficulty Heraclitus sees of interpreting meaning in the world in general, as E. L. Hussey remarks: 'The "meaning of the world", like that of a statement in words, is not obvious, but yet is present in the statement, and can be worked out provided one "knows the language".'[16] In other words, this fragment could be said to enact, rather than simply describe, the relationship between mortality and immortality, life and death; i.e., one that is difficult to discern and which rests on the possibility that there may not be much between them.[17]

The work of the author of *On Breaths* does not, of course, directly broach such a topic as 'the meaning of the world' but, as we saw above in the comparison with Gorgias' *Encomium of Helen*, he does employ play on sound to embody his understanding of aspects of nature in a way that is strikingly reminiscent of Heraclitus' use of language. Play on the arrangement of words and syntax is very common in *On Breaths* as in, for instance, 'πλησμονὴν ἰᾶται κένωσις, κένωσιν δὲ πλησμονή, πόνον δὲ ἀπονίη, ἀπονίην δὲ πόνος' 'excess is cured by emptying, emptiness by excess, work by rest, rest by work' (*On Breaths*, 1.4). The placement of words in a succinct list and use of an 'a-b, b-a' structure that involves repetition of words and therefore of sounds does not merely explain how oppositions are important to medicine but reflects their importance – their nature even – by communicating a neat and concise rhythm and structure that reflects the concise relationship that the author claims is in the nature of medicine.

Similarly, the author of *On the Sacred Disease* also uses the arrangement of words and repetition of sounds to express his understanding of the nature of human physical constitutions and disease transmission. He states 'ἐκ τοῦ φλεγματώδεος φλεγματώδης, καὶ ἐκ χολώδεος χολώδης γίνεται, καὶ ἐκ φθινώδεος φθινώδης, καὶ ἐκ σπληνώδεος σπληνίης' 'a phlegmatic [parent] has a phlegmatic [child], a bilious [parent] a bilious [child], a consumptive [parent] a consumptive [child], and a splenetic [parent] a splenetic [child]' (*On the Sacred Disease*, 2.2). The use of *polyptoton* here (repeating the same word with a different inflexion) embodies the notion of generation – that like generates like – which is central to the author's account of the 'sacred' disease.[18]

As well as these more straightforward examples of patterning in sound and structure, we also find more elaborate examples of patterning in *On Breaths*, many of which reflect the elaborate use of sound patterning found in Heraclitus, as in the following example, which discusses a principle of the nature of diseases:

> Τῶν δὲ δὴ νούσων ἁπασέων ὁ μὲν τρόπος ωὑτός, ὁ δὲ τόπος διαφέρει. Δοκεῖ μὲν οὖν οὐδὲν ἐοικέναι τὰ νοσήματα ἀλλήλοισιν διὰ τὴν ἀλλοιότητα τῶν τόπων, ἔστι δὲ μία πασέων νούσων καὶ ἰδέη καὶ αἰτίη ἡ αὐτή.

> Of all diseases the character is the same, but the seat varies. So while diseases are thought to be entirely unlike one another, owing to the difference in their seat, in reality all have one essence and cause.
>
> *(On Breaths, 2.1)*

The words 'τρόπος' 'way' or 'type' and 'τόπος' 'place' mimic the contrast that is made between sameness and difference in the statement, for these two words are almost identical in spelling but differ widely in their field of reference: the author uses play on slight variation in sound to underline the idea that diseases can be the same in one aspect ('τρόπος' and 'τόπος' sound almost the same) but different in another ('τρόπος' and 'τόπος' have very different meanings). The author then goes on to state that these diseases seem to be in no way like 'one another' ('ἀλλήλων') because of the 'difference' ('ἀλλοιότητος') of place. These two key words in the sentence are similar in sound, for they share the same first syllable 'ἀλλ' and the similar, probably /aʊ/ and /ɔɪ/ sounds corresponding to 'ω' in the former case and 'οι' in the latter. So, the similarity in sound contrasts with their difference in meaning and echoes the overall point being made in the sentence: that all diseases are the same despite apparent differences.

The idea of one thing – in this case the 'τρόπος' ('character') of diseases – having different aspects – in this case the 'τόπος' ('seat') of diseases – recalls Heraclitus' use of sound in the following fragment, where Heraclitus exploits sound to stress the epistemological point he is making.

> θάλασσα ὕδωρ καθαρώτατον καὶ μιαρώτατον· ἰχθύσι μὲν πότιμον καὶ σωτήριον, ἀνθρώποις δὲ ἄποτον καὶ ὀλέθριον.

> Sea is the purest and most polluted water: for fish drinkable and healthy; for people undrinkable and harmful.[19]

Here, we are presented with the notion that different forms of life experience the same thing in an opposite fashion: sea water is the same for both humans and sea fish in that it is sea water, but their experience of sea water can be said to be opposite, for it allows sea fish to live and can kill humans if consumed. The opposition in the fragment from Heraclitus is highlighted through the use of repetition of sound: the ending of the superlative adjectives '-ώτατον' helps to underline the idea that these two adjectives are describing the same noun; the use of the superlative adjective rather than the positive form emphasises the extreme difference in experience each adjective represents. The sounds 'ποτ' and 'ον' in the words 'πότιμον' and 'ἄποτον' also help to highlight the idea that both adjectives are used to describe sea water. Here, as we saw in the passage mentioned above, Heraclitus states an opposition only to undermine it.

Another close parallel to the example from *On Breaths* above is in Heraclitus' famous aphorism that declares that one cannot step into the same river twice:

> ποταμοῖσι τοῖσιν αὐτοῖσιν ἐμβαίνουσιν ἕτερα καὶ ἕτερα ὕδατα ἐπιρρεῖ.

> On those stepping into rivers staying the same other and other waters flow.[20]

Here the similar-sounding '-οισι', '-οισιν' and '-ούσιν' and the repetition of the word 'ἕτερα' 'others' highlights the delicate contrast – even ambiguity or paradox – between the idea of the 'same' rivers and the continually changing waters. The Heraclitean example is even more succinct and effective than the examples from *On Breaths* at collapsing the distinction between sameness and difference through play on sound.

Another case of repetition of sounds in *On Breaths* used to echo a contrast between notions of sameness and difference is found following the author's definition of epidemic fever, where the author qualifies the idea that fever is the same for all with the following account:

> διαφέρει . . . καὶ σῶμα σώματος καὶ φύσις φύσιος καὶ τροφὴ τροφῆς. οὐ γὰρ πᾶσι τοῖσιν ἔθνεσιν τῶν ζῴων ταὐτὰ οὔτ' ἀνάρμοστα οὔτ' εὐάρμοστά ἐστιν, ἀλλ' ἕτερα ἑτέροισι σύμφορα καὶ ἕτερα ἑτέροισιν ἀσύμφορα.

> one body differs from another, one nature from another and one nutriment from another. For the same things are not inappropriate nor appropriate for all types of living being, but some are useful for some and some are harmful to some.

> (*On Breaths*, 6.2)

The three key nouns here are in different cases (nominative and genitive singular respectively); the grammatical morphology means that there is a difference in spelling between the nominative and the genitive which reflects the conceptual difference that the author wishes to express while the fact that the same word is repeated reflects the standard assumption, which the author claims is insufficiently nuanced, that bodies, natures and nutriments are all the same. The underlying rhetorical device is that small similarities and differences in orthography are being exploited to underline the general concept that apparent similarity does not preclude differences.

The following sentence, discussed in the previous chapter as an illustration of the dense use of oppositions, also forms part of an example of what Kahn (1979), discussing Heraclitus, would call resonance, which is phonetic in terms of the presence of an identifiable rhythm:

> ὁ γὰρ βίος μεταβολέων πλέος· τοῦτο δὲ μοῦνον ἀεὶ διατελέουσιν ἅπαντα τὰ θνητὰ ζῷα πρήσσοντα, τοτὲ μὲν ἐμπνέοντα, τοτὲ δὲ ἀναπνέοντα.

> for life is full of changes; but breathing alone is continuous for all living beings, inspiration and expiration being alternate.
>
> (*On Breaths*, 4.3)

The phrase 'τοτὲ μὲν ἐμπνέοντα, τοτὲ δὲ ἀναπνέοντα', which literally means 'now breathing in, now breathing out' and which mimics the action that is being described, is then echoed in rhythm and in the contrast between movement 'in' and movement 'out' several lines later in the treatise in the phrase 'ἐπιδείξω τὰ νοσήματα τούτου ἀπόγονά τε καὶ ἔκγονα πάντα ἐόντα.' 'I will show that diseases all come from things coming to and going from the body' (*On Breaths*, 5.2). By 'ἀπόγονά τε καὶ ἔκγονα' 'things coming to and going from the body', the author means air, as he goes on to make clear in the discussion of types of fever in Sections 6 and 7 which follow immediately after this. The resonance is subtle, but it nevertheless helps to build up the coherency of the account and to insist on the primacy of air in disease causation.

The use of resonance in Heraclitus, as we saw in the example of the repetition of the word 'βίος', gives the author the opportunity to develop further the pun that has already been made. In *On Breaths*, by contrast, the phonetic resonance is used to build up correspondence between different parts of the account but is not in itself developed further.

*

To draw some conclusions, we have seen how in both Gorgias' *Encomium of Helen* and in the Hippocratic *On Breaths* structure of phrasing embodies in many cases the message that is being communicated. In both treatises, we find examples of oppositions described in the text being used as support for a broader generalisation. We have seen how the neatness of the oppositions – the sense that they are black and white – endows the generalisations made with a sense of neatness and 'fit'. We have also seen how word play is used in both treatises; there is a certain amount of overlap but this does not feed directly into the relationship between form and content in the treatises.

It is also clear that we find a somewhat different relationship to language and argument in *Encomium of Helen* from *On Breaths*, with the former being a mock defence and the latter possibly being a more serious contribution to medicine and containing word play that is beyond the scope of what we find in *Encomium of Helen*. We also find a range of examples of repetition of sounds and phrases in *On Breaths* that have no parallel in *Encomium of Helen*, as in the repetition of certain similar-sounding words for emphasising a point and the repetition of words in order to demarcate the stages in a process.

In examining the relationship between Heraclitus' work and *On Breaths*, we have seen that there are examples of phrases enacting ideas in both, as in Gorgias' *Encomium of Helen*. Specific to the contrast between Heraclitus and *On Breaths*, however, is the way that small similarities and differences in orthography are exploited to convey a sense of *both* similarity *and* difference simultaneously. We also find some sense of resonance in *On Breaths* that is reminiscent of the same in Heraclitus.

We cannot know for sure that the connection between the author of *On Breaths* and *Encomium of Helen* or between *On Breaths* and Heraclitus was a direct one, but there certainly is evidence of a very strong link between the two authors and a specific influence in terms of the use of sound. That *On the Sacred Disease* shows much less influence fits in with the idea that there was a variety of ways of writing persuasively which were being explored in the fifth and early fourth centuries BCE.

Notes

1 'aucune œuvre, dans la littérature conservée, n'est aussi proche de l'*Éloge d'Hélène* que le traité des *Vents*.'
2 'La principale caractéristique du style périodique est l'emploi de l'antithèse qui oppose deux membres de phrase de même longueur (parisose) se terminant par les memes sonorities (paromoiose).'
3 cf. Aristotle, *Rhetoric,* III, 1, 1404a25.
4 'plusieurs de ces images puisent-elles leur source première dans la prose technique ionienne qui semble naturellement imagée et dont la coloration dite poétique vient peut-être moins de l'imitation de la poésie (épique, lyrique ou tragique) que de la richesse d'un fonds ionien commun à la prose et à la poésie.'
5 E.g. 'ἀφανεστάτων καὶ χαλεπωτάτων' in *On Breaths*, 1, 103, 10f.
6 'la reprise d'un même terme pour relier les phrases entre elles et pour marquer les étapes d'un raissonement et d'un processus physiologique, comme en c.14, 122, 1 ψύχθέντι δὲ τῷ αἴματι reprend τὸ αἷμα ψύχεται, est une caractéristique de la prose ionienne qui n'a pas subi l'influence de la sophistique.'
7 Lausberg (1998) describes parechema as a special case of *annominatio* (see §1246, under paréchème); for *annominatio* see §§637–639.

 8 For further information on the term 'homonym' see Lausberg (1998: 877) '*Rhetoric*' under '*homonyme*'.
 9 For an overview of Heraclitus' work, see e.g. Graham (2008: 169–188) and Barnes (1979: 57–81).
10 See Jones (1998–2005 [1923–1931], vol. I: xxiv–xxvi).
11 Gorgias' interest in the potential ambiguity of language and his interest in its connection with nature is one general area of influence of Heraclitus, as M. Untersteiner points out (1954: 106–107).
12 Kahn 1979: 87-95 and *passim*. Famous examples of Heraclitus' use of punning which also show syntactic play and resonance include the following. 'βιός τῷ τόξῳ ὄνομα βίος, ἔργον δὲ θάνατος' 'The name of the bow is life; its work is death' [DK22B48] plays on the double meaning of 'βίος' as 'life' and 'βιός' as 'bow'). In the maxim 'ταὐτό τ᾽ ἔνι ζῶν καὶ τεθνηκὸς καὶ τὸ ἐγρηγορὸς καὶ καθεῦδον καὶ νέον καὶ γηραιόν· τάδε γὰρ μεταπεσόντα ἐκεῖνά ἐστι κἀκεῖνα [πάλιν] μεταπεσόντα ταῦτα' 'The same . . . : living and dead, and the waking and the sleeping, and young and old. For these transposed are those, and those transposed again are these' [DK22B88], the ambiguity of the words 'τάδε' 'these' (here), 'ἐκεῖνα' 'those' and 'ταῦτα' 'these' (here) is prominent; and we saw 'οὐ ξυνιᾶσιν ὅκως διαφερόμενον ἑωυτῷ ξυμφέρεται· παλίντονος ἁρμονίη ὅκωσπερ τόξου καὶ λύρης' 'They do not comprehend how a thing agrees at variance with itself; it is an attunement turning back on itself, like that of the bow and the lyre' [DK22B51] which picks up on and develops the pun on 'βίος' in the first example above and shows resonance between the fragments.
13 DK22B1 (cited in Sextus Empiricus *Against the Professors* and Hippolytus *Refutation*).
14 DK22B62 (cited in Hippolytus); see also Graham (2010: 169, citation 112).
15 The theme of a quest for understanding is picked up on in other fragments, such as 'ἐδιζησάμην ἐμεωυτόν' 'I inquired of myself' (DK22B101 (cited in Plutarch *Against Colotes*); see also: Graham, 2010: 149, citation 38)) and 'ἀνθρώποισι πᾶσι μέτεστι γινώσκειν ἑωυτοὺς καὶ σωφρονεῖν' 'It belongs to all men to know themselves and to think well' (DK22B116 (cited in Stobaeus); see also: Graham, 2010: 147, citation 30).
16 See Honderich (1995: 351–352). For a more detailed analysis of Heraclitus' epistemology see Hussey (1982: 33–59).
17 Kahn (1979: 124) notes: 'It is not that reality as such is contradictory; what is reflected in the semantic difficulty of interpreting these utterances is the epistemic difficulty of grasping such a structure, the cosmic *logos*, as the underlying unity for our own experience of opposition and contrast.' Kahn also notes that 'the doctrine of unity or interdependence between opposing powers . . . constitutes the general pattern and the formal theme for Heraclitus' teaching' (1979: 109).
18 For the term *polyptoton* see Lausberg (1998: 288–291).
19 DK22B61 (cited in Hippolytus *Refutation*); see also Graham (2010: 163, citation 79).
20 DK22B12 (cited in Eusebius *Preparation for the Gospel* and Arius Didymus); see also Graham (2010: 159, citation 62).

References

Barnes, J. (1979), *The Presocratic Philosophers. Vol.1, Thales to Zeno*. London: Routledge and Kegan Paul. 57–81.

Graham, D. W. (2010), *The Texts of Early Greek Philosophy: The Complete Fragments and Selected Testimonies of the Major Presocratics*. Cambridge: Cambridge University Press.

Graham, D. W. (2008), 'Heraclitus: Flux, Order and Knowledge' in Curd, P. and Graham, D. W. (eds.), *The Oxford Handbook of Presocratic Philosophy*. Oxford: Oxford University Press. 169–188.

Honderich, T. (ed.) (1995), *The Oxford Companion to Philosophy*. Oxford: Oxford University Press.

Hussey, E. (1982), 'Epistemology and Meaning in Heraclitus' in Schofield, M. and Nussbaum, M. (eds.), *Language and Logos: Studies in Ancient Greek Philosophy Presented to G. E. L. Owen*. Cambridge; New York: Cambridge University Press. 33–59.

Jones, W. H. S. (ed. and trans.) (1998–2005 [1923–1931]), *Hippocrates I–IV*. Cambridge, MA; London: Harvard University Press.

Jouanna, J. (ed. and trans.) (1988), *Hippocrate. Tome V, 1re partie. Des vents; De l'art*. Paris: Les Belles Lettres.

Jouanna, J. (1984), 'Rhétorique et médecine dans la collection Hippocratique: contribution à l'histoire de la rhétorique au Ve siècle.' *Revue des Études greques* 97. Paris: Société d'Edition 'Les Belles Lettres'. 26–44.

Kahn, C. H. (1979), *The Art and Thought of Heraclitus: An Edition of the Fragments with Translation and Commentary*. Cambridge; New York: Cambridge University Press.

Lausberg, H. (1998), *Handbook of Literary Rhetoric: A Foundation for Literary Study*; translated by M. T. Bliss, A. Jansen, and D. E. Orton; edited by D. E. Orton and R. D. Anderson. Leiden; Boston, MA: Brill.

Untersteiner, M. (1954), *The Sophists*; translated by K. Freeman. Oxford: Blackwell.

Waterfield, R. (2009 [2000]), *The First Philosophers: The Presocratics and the Sophists*. Oxford: Oxford University Press.

5 In the *agon*: the persuasive functions of antithesis in Hippocratic oratory

In the previous chapter, on the connections between sound play and meaning in *On Breaths* and models for this, we saw how the sound of words and rhythm are used in the example of Hippocratic oratory to echo, enhance and embody important ideas which the authors wish to communicate, and how this use of sound can be traced back to Heraclitus' intricately composed philosophical maxims, which embrace ambiguity of reference and phonic play to establish a philosophical point, and to Gorgias' *Helen*, which also makes use of sound and rhythm to convey layers of meaning beyond the surface content of phrases and sentences.

In this chapter, I turn to an analysis of the use of antithesis in Hippocratic expository prose. There are many indications at all levels of cultural activity that ancient Greeks tended to view the world in conflictual terms. The binary opposition between Greek-speakers and barbarians is one example of this; the way in which communities established their identities by defining the 'other' – what they are not – is a topic which has been the subject of several recent studies, for instance Edith Hall's *Inventing the Barbarian* (1989) and which we can see played out again and again in Greek literature, including, for example, the Hippocratic treatise *Airs, Waters, Places*, which deals with 'opposite' climatic conditions and locations in the first half, and with dichotomised differences between European and Asiatic cultures in the second half.[1] As has already been noted in Chapter 2, Hankinson finds an allopathic principle underlying Hippocratic medicine in *On the Sacred Disease*, that opposites cure opposites, which is also reflected in the famous theory of humours as most explicitly stated in *On the Nature of Human Beings* (4.1). At the level of prose composition too, the use of oppositional structures, for example the 'μὲν . . . δέ' 'on the one hand . . . on the other hand' construction is a fundamental building block of the language.

This chapter is concerned with the various ways in which antitheses are prominent in the Hippocratic oratorical treatises and their persuasive function. The chapter focuses on how antitheses in these writings are employed to establish boundaries of authority and to acknowledge and emphasise the drama of the competitive oratorical context for which they were likely to have been composed. It will also be argued that the accumulation of antithetical pairs establishes a relationship and hierarchy between the speaker and the audience and/or opponents; identifies parameters in which a theory can be judged; and communicates underlying moral messages to the audience which may go beyond the realms of medical debate.

There is some scholarly work on this subject in the context of the Hippocratic Collection, most notably Geoffrey Lloyd's *Polarity and Analogy*. In this volume, Lloyd includes a survey of theories based on opposites in ancient Greek thought – including, for instance, Anaximander's and Heraclitus' ideas about the unity of opposites – and then goes on to establish distinct categories in logical argument. This latter approach is inspired in part by Aristotle's analysis of oppositional relations between terms. Following Aristotle in *Prior Analytics* and *On Interpretation*, Lloyd notes, for instance, that 'The English terms 'opposite' and 'opposition', like the Greek ἀντικείμενον and ἀντικεῖσθαι, are used to refer to many different types of relationship' (Lloyd 1966: 86 f.) and traces the establishment of logical oppositions from Parmenides onwards in early Greek thought, assessing their logical validity. Lloyd notes that

> Certain criticisms apply to the majority of the arguments which we have considered [from the Platonic period]. (1) It was generally the case that the terms used in such arguments were quite equivocal, e.g. 'it is', 'the many'. (2) It seems that certain 'hypotheses' were often treated as though, like propositions, they must be either true or false. (3) The relationships between opposites of different sorts were evidently sometimes misconceived or oversimplified.
>
> (1966: 126)

Lloyd accounts, then, for the philosophically logical quality of opposition, but is less concerned with its persuasive function, though, as argued in Chapters 3 and 4 above, it would seem that persuasion through patterning was an important attribute of the truth value of early Greek prose.

Other scholars have used a similar approach to Lloyd's as a basis for interpretation of Hippocratic treatises. M. Fantuzzi, for example, notes of *On Ancient Medicine*:

> the conscious reuse of polar thinking in *On Ancient Medicine* can be treated as a system of logic. Beyond formal syllogistic structures, the simple phrasal movement playing out between synonymous and antithetical pairs sets up parallels and examples of *chiasmus*, suggesting through their paths indirect connections.
>
> (1983: 242)[2]

For Fantuzzi, then, the abundance of oppositional structures in *On Ancient Medicine*, though not in the form of formal syllogisms, does suggest systematic, philosophically logical thinking. Jane Barton also discusses explanation in *On Ancient Medicine* and claims that the author of the treatise defends inductive inference as the means by which medical research proceeds as opposed to deductive inference in philosophy (2005: esp. 43–44).

This chapter seeks to offer a fresh reading of use of antitheses which examines them as both boundary setting and conveying subtle meanings through association, rather than through the lens of philosophical logic, for reasons outlined in the preceding chapters of this book. This kind of reading is modelled most closely on Charles Kahn's approach to Heraclitus' work (1979); no study of chains of associations and patterns in the Hippocratic Collection has, to my knowledge, been carried out so far.

In the first part of this chapter, I examine the range of functions of some of the most striking uses of opposition and clusters of oppositional phrases in *On Breaths*, *On the Art*, *On Ancient Medicine*, *On the Nature of Human Beings* and *On the Sacred Disease*. In each of the five treatises, I examine the persuasive function of oppositional formulae and consider how form and content relate to one another in such instances to communicate various layers of meaning beyond the more obvious surface content. Frequently, clusters of oppositional pairs are found at or near the beginning of treatises and seem to serve to establish a conceptual framework through which other ideas in the treatise can be conveyed.

In the second part of this chapter, I analyse in further detail associations between oppositional pairs in *On Ancient Medicine*, where there is a more elaborate level of patterning than in the other Hippocratic treatises examined and a richer set of resonances and implied meanings is to be found.

In the third part of the chapter, I consider further the evidence for associations of oppositions in *On the Sacred Disease*, in light of the attention to the persuasive strategies this treatise in particular has been given in scholarship. I explore in detail how my reading of associations between oppositional constructions complements the work of Philip van der Eijk and Julie Laskaris on this treatise by highlighting the relevance of acknowledging associations between oppositional constructions in appreciating the consistency of the treatise.

The persuasive function of oppositions in Hippocratic oratorical treatises

(a) On Breaths

On Breaths opens with a series of general statements on the nature of the medical art, the work of the physician and the role of medicine in healing, and points out repeatedly the distance in terms of knowledge and experience between the physician and the layperson. Medicine is said to be a burden for those who are initiated into it, yet a source of help to those who benefit from it. Medicine is introduced as a 'τέχνη' in the context of Greek intellectual categorisation: 'Τῶν δὲ δὴ τοιούτων ἐστὶν τεχνέων . . . ἣν οἱ Ἕλληνες καλέουσιν ἰητρικήν' 'Of such arts there is one which the Greeks call medicine' (1.2). Medicine is said to oppose those things – illness, disease, suffering, death – that are bad in life (1.2). The author also states that 'τὰ μὲν φλαῦρα χαλεπὸν γνῶναι, τὰ δὲ σπουδαῖα ῥηΐδιον' 'The bad aspects [of the art] are difficult to understand while the good aspects are easy to comprehend' (1.3). A further distinction is drawn here between the relative success of intellectual understanding and manual skill in dealing with complex medical problems (1.3).

As well as these oppositions between good and bad and between intellect and manual skill, opposition is expressed through rhetorical call and response in the opening of *On Breaths*, as in the following: 'Τί οὖν λιμοῦ φάρμακον; Ὃ παύει λιμόν' 'What then is the remedy for hunger? That which makes hunger cease' (1.4) where we find the antithesis between being hungry and not being hungry. We also find two antithetical pairs linked in an a-b, b-a structure in the following example. In the phrase 'τοῖσι μὲν κεκτημένοισίν εἰσιν ἐπίπονοι, τοῖσι δὲ χρεωμένοισιν ὀνήϊστοι, καὶ τοῖσι μὲν δημότῃσιν ξυνὸν ἀγαθόν, τοῖσι δὲ μεταχειπιζομένοισί σφας λυπηραί.' 'to those that possess them they are painful, but to those that use them are helpful, a common good to laymen, but to those that practise them grievous.' (1.1) the second antithesis is inverted so that we have the structure 'pain/ benefit; common good/grief'.[3]

The principal oppositions in use in 1.1–1.5 can be listed as follows, relating to two main strands – the distinction between the doctor and the layperson and oppositions relating to the balance needed for health (see Tables 5.1 and 5.2 on the following page).

The first cluster of oppositional pairs serves to attract attention to the speaker and add drama to the delivery of the introduction of the topic of discussion; to establish authority by stipulating a hierarchy of expertise and other social distinctions, and, linked to this, to signal association with models of a defence of the art commonly circulating in this period.

The generalising, confident sweep of both sets of oppositions also serves to establish the authority and grasp of the voice 'speaking' to us and pave the way for an explanation of disease that will itself trade heavily on antithetical substances/qualities/forces. On this latter point, the author notes 'τὰ ἐναντία τῶν ἐναντίων ἐστὶν ἰήματα' 'opposites are cures for opposites' (1.5) a phrase which describes an allopathic principle of medicine that underlines the medical explanations that the author presents here and that chimes with his tendency to use antithetical expressions at this point in the text.

Table 5.1 Oppositions relating to the distinction between the doctor and the layperson in *On Breaths* 1.1–3; 1.5[4]

experiencing pain as a consequence of possessing the art	experiencing benefit or relief as a consequence of using the art
a grievance to doctors	a common good
difficulty of understanding bad aspects	ease of understanding good aspects
experience	inexperience
best physician	worst physician

Table 5.2 Oppositions relating to the balance needed for health in *On Breaths* 1.4–5[5]

hunger	consuming food
thirst	consuming liquid
depletion	repletion
rest	exercise
subtraction	addition
lack	excess

(b) On Ancient Medicine

Just as in *On Breaths*, the opening section of *On Ancient Medicine* employs a high number of oppositional pairings which relate to the social distinctions and hierarchies of medical practitioners. As with the oppositions employed in the opening of *On Breaths*, many serve to attract attention and dramatise the discussion as agonistic, as well as establishing parameters for the author's account to follow.

The treatise begins by claiming that those who have spoken or written about medicine 'basing their account on one or two primary elements or causes' are erroneous in their analysis and should be blamed because the art of medicine in fact exists and has craftsmen and practitioners who are held in esteem (1.1). It also asserts that while some practitioners are bad and others good, medicine has no need of a novel hypothesis as obscure and dubious matters have (1.2–3). The author admits that it is necessary to develop a new hypothesis about things in the sky or under the earth, but notes that it would not be possible to check whether such hypotheses were true or false, and obtain clear knowledge, unlike the case for medicine (1.3).

While some of the oppositions are mere alternatives – for example, Ὁκόσοι ἐπεχείρησαν περὶ ἰητρικῆς λέγειν ἢ γράφειν 'All those who have undertaken to speak or write about medicine' (1.1) and 'ἓν ἢ δύο ὑποθέμενοι' 'one or two hypotheses' (1.1) others are closer to black-and-white dichotomies, such as 'Εἰσὶ δὲ δημιουργοὶ οἱ μὲν φλαῦροι, οἱ δὲ πολλὸν διαφέροντες' 'Some practitioners are bad, while others are much better' (1.2).

The overall aim of the author in this opening section is to indicate a boundary between what can be known for certain and what cannot: 'εἴτε ἀληθέα ἐστὶν εἴτε μή' 'whether what [the speaker] says is true or not' (1.3) and the distinction between what is knowable and what is not, implied in 'Διὸ οὐκ ἠξίουν αὐτὴν ἔγωγε καινῆς ὑποθέσιος δεῖσθαι, ὥσπερ τὰ ἀφανέα τε καὶ ἀπορεόμενα' 'For this reason I have deemed that medicine has no need of a newfangled hypothesis, as do obscure and dubious matters' (1.3). By repeating the point that some things are true and others not, and that some things are knowable and others not, the author establishes a clear position in relation to his opponents. The accumulation of such oppositional pairs renders the antagonistic attitude to his opponents more emphatic.

We also find evidence of word patterning in the first section of the treatise in the following: 'ὑπόθεσιν αὐτοὶ ἑωυτοῖσιν ὑποθέμενοι' 'having laid down as a hypothesis for their account' (1.1), showing an a-b-b-a structure, which may reflect the point that the author is making that the medical innovators are entangled in their own rhetoric. Having said this, his description of the technique of the medical innovators 'ἐς βραχὺ ἄγοντες τὴν ἀρχὴν τῆς αἰτίης τοῖσιν ἀνθρώποισι τῶν νούσων τε καὶ τοῦ θανάτου' 'narrowing down the primary cause of diseases or death for human beings' (1.1) in one sense reflects this author's own approach in *excluding* the possibility that the origin of the cause of diseases could be one element or principle: in other words, he applies 'either / or' statements to the ideas of the medical innovators in the same way that they are characterised as applying exclusive categories to the origins of medicine. Indeed, the fundamental dichotomy traded on in this section is that between the old ways and medical innovation. Medical innovation is here characterised, therefore, and maintains its upper hand over the old ways, through insistence on binary opposites.

The principal sense here of binary opposition between the author and his methods and views and his opponents' and theirs is further entrenched with the use of moralising language by the author. The uses the verbs 'ἁμαρτάνω', 'to fail' (1.1) to describe the error of their approach and 'μέμφομαι' 'to blame' (1.1) to indicate an appropriate response.[6] This gives the impression of the medical innovators being publically judged and shamed. The references to 'τοῖσι μεγίστοισι' 'in the most important circumstances' and 'τιμῶσι μάλιστα' 'hold in special honour' in the sentence 'μάλιστα δὲ ἄξιον μέμψασθαι, ὅτι ἀμφὶ τέχνης ἐούσης ᾗ χρέονταί τε πάντες ἐπὶ τοῖσι μεγίστοισι καὶ τιμῶσι μάλιστα τοὺς ἀγαθοὺς χειροτέχνας καὶ δημιουργούς' 'But as they are especially worthy of blame because their errors concern an art that really exists, one which all people make use of in the most important circumstances and whose good craftsmen and practitioners all hold in special honour' (1.1) further enhance this ambience of praise and blame and of honour, which is linked by association to the contrast between truth and falsehood.

The author's persuasive strategy trades in grand and general truths about the origin of the causes of diseases, about how the medical innovators make claims about medicine, about the general use of medicine and in characterising what is *not* the case about medicine, both in terms of general knowledge about medicine and about the progress that has been made in learning about medicine up to this point in time. Many of these instances of the term 'πᾶς' are used to emphasise what all people have in common, and therefore to convey a sense of a speaker who speaks for the common good, with the medical innovators characterised as outsiders.

The author also explicitly refers to his interest in and technique of differentiation between extremes: the term 'πολλόν' 'much' and the verb 'διαφέρω' 'differ' echoing in both the following phrases 'Εἰσὶ δὲ δημιουργοὶ οἱ μὲν φλαῦροι, οἱ δὲ πολλὸν διαφέροντες' 'Some practitioners are bad, while others are much better' (1.2) and 'οἱ δημιουργοὶ πολλὸν ἀλλήλων διαφέρουσι κατὰ χεῖρα καὶ κατὰ γνώμην' 'practitioners differ greatly from one another in manual skill and judgement' (1.2); the emphasis on extreme degrees of difference, which essentially equates to further oppositional pairs, also helps the author establish memorable grand and general truths.

These oppositions show a strong concern to establish the intellectual and moral high ground. As with *On Breaths*, the association between pairs of oppositions – for example between truth and falsehood and the old medical ways and medical innovation – help to establish a network of underlying meanings that the author can then develop further in the remainder of the treatise. The use of oppositions is more complex than in *On Breaths*, with listing, complementary pairs and added moralising vocabulary employed. Nonetheless, it is clear that the oppositions serve a dramatic function to cast the speaker in a heroic light and undermine the opponents; it is also clear that part of the persuasive strategy of the author is to establish precedence by the use of binary pairs as well as other rhetorical strategies: the *singleness* of the opponents' theory is ridiculed in favour of a theoretical position that is conveyed in a range of binary and listing forms. This is to say that the *way* in which the theory is expressed carries a great deal of force in the absence of any other means of proving that one theory is truer than another.

Overall, the opening conveys a certain anxiety about false reasoning and claims a moral high ground in approaching the subject. The opening implies a contest between truth and falsehood, and between tried and tested ways of reasoning and medical innovation. The author is also concerned about quality assurance, about celebrating progress in medical knowledge, and about making clear certain boundaries between what is and what is known, and about proper and improper methodology. There is also, arguably, the sense that the author is trying to rescue medicine from slander, appealing to the common knowledge of all people and against obfuscation and trickery. The author's rhetoric is forceful, repetitive, intricate and controlling.

The references to 'Ὁκόσοι ἐπεχείρησαν περὶ ἰητρικῆς λέγειν ἢ γράφειν' 'All those who have undertaken to speak or to write about medicine' (1.1) and 'ἄλλο τι ἂν θέλωσιν' 'anything else they want' (1.1) and 'οἷον περὶ τῶν μετεώρων ἢ τῶν ὑπὸ γῆν· ἅ εἰ τις λέγοι καὶ γινώσκοι ὡς ἔχει' 'about things in the sky or under the earth: if anyone should recognise and state how these things are' (1.3) imply absence of standards by which expertise can be measured. This could go some way to explain the author's apparent anxiety about needing to establish standards of practice and points of truth.

(c) On the Sacred Disease

The use of oppositional pairing in the opening of *On the Sacred Disease* is somewhat less obvious and emphatic than in either *On Breaths* or *On Ancient Medicine*; the prologue is also lengthier and more complex and detailed than in these other treatises. Oppositional pairs are present, nonetheless, and refer to the distinction between the speaker and his opponents as well as to the core of the author's argument.

The argument of the opening is constructed on a series of binary oppositions: between what is sacred and what is not; between the 'professional' doctor and the imposters; between one sacred disease and many; between Libyans and Greeks; and between piety and impiety. The use of one further binary opposition – between becoming ensnarled in a problem and finding its solution – is underlined in the language used by the author:

> Καὶ κατὰ μὲν τὴν ἀπορίην αὐτοῖσι τοῦ μὴ γινώσκειν τὸ θεῖον αὐτῇ διασώζεται, κατὰ δὲ τὴν εὐπορίην τοῦ τρόπου τῆς ἰήσιος ᾧ ἰῶνται, ἀπόλλυται, ὅτι καθαρμοῖσί τε ἰῶνται καὶ ἐπαοιδῇσιν.

> In virtue of their inability to understand it, the divine character of the disease is preserved, but in virtue of the ease of the manner of cure that they employ it disappears, in that they cure it by purifications and incantations.
>
> (*On the Sacred Disease*, 1.2)

The pair 'ἀπορίην . . . εὐπορίην' 'inability . . . ability' pinpoints the contrast of the sentence here and also sums up the general point being made in this first section of the treatise: that the healers seem very able but in fact cover up their lack of knowledge. The comparison is a subtle one, and the similarity of the two words in Greek reflects the subtlety of the distinction being made here.

The subtle opposition expressed in the words 'ἀπορίην . . . εὐπορίην' is echoed and further developed later in the section:

> Καίτοι ἔμοιγε οὐ περὶ εὐσεβείης δοκέουσι τοὺς λόγους ποιεῖσθαι, ὡς οἴονται, ἀλλὰ περὶ δυσσεβείης μᾶλλον καὶ ὡς οἱ θεοὶ οὐκ εἰσί· τό τε εὐσεβὲς αὐτῶν καὶ θεῖον ἀσεβές καὶ ἀνόσιόν ἐστιν, ὡς ἐγὼ διδάξω.

> Moreover, as I think, their discussions are not focused on piety, as they imagine, but rather on impiety and on the idea that the gods do not exist. Their conception of what is pious and the divine is in reality impious and sacrilegious, as I will show.
>
> (*On the Sacred Disease*, 1.8)

Here the contrast between the words 'εὐσεβείης' 'piety' and 'δυσσεβείης' 'impiety' and between 'εὐσεβὲς' 'pious' and 'ἀσεβὲς' impious helps to underscore the point being made: the close similarity between these words in terms of their spelling helps to emphasise the subtlety of the point that the author is making here and hint at the difficulty of making such distinctions.

We also find the author making use of generalising terms to refer to the activities of his opponents along with an accumulation of repeated negatives to frame his attack; this has the effect of dramatising the nature of the disagreement between them and sets up a binary argument over ambitious claims to knowledge:

> Εἰ γὰρ σελήνην τε καθαιρεῖν καὶ ἥλιον ἀφανίζειν καὶ χειμῶνά τε καὶ εὐδίην ποιεῖν καὶ ὄμβρους καὶ αὐχμοὺς καὶ θάλασσαν ἄφορον καὶ γῆν καὶ τἆλλα τὰ τοιουτότροπα πάντα ὑποδέχονται ἐπίστασθαι – εἴτε καὶ ἐκ τελετέων εἴτε καὶ ἐξ ἄλλης τινὸς γνώμης ἢ μελέτης φασὶ ταῦτα οἷόν τ' εἶναι γενέσθαι – οἱ ταῦτ' ἐπιτηδεύοντες δύσσεβεῖν ἔμοιγε δοκέουσι καὶ θεοὺς οὔτε εἶναι νομίζειν οὔτε ἰσχύειν οὐδὲν, οὔτ' εἴργεσθαι ἂν οὐδενὸς τῶν ἐσχάτων ποιέοντες, ὡς οὐ δεινοὶ αὐτοῖσίν εἰσιν;

> For if they profess to know how to bring down the moon, to eclipse the sun, to make storm and sunshine, rain and drought, the sea impassable and the earth barren, and all other such wonders – whether it be by rites or by some cunning or practice that they can affirm these prodigies possible – in any case I am sure that they are impious, and cannot believe that the gods exist or have any strength, and that they would not refrain from the most extreme actions, since the gods surely do not seem terrible to them.
>
> (*On the Sacred Disease*, 1.9)

In the quotation, the author uses an accumulated list of items to characterise his opponents' professed areas of knowledge, which culminates in a generalising tag – 'καὶ τἆλλα τὰ τοιουτότροπα πάντα' 'and all other such [wonders]' – which implies that the opponents lay claim to a full understanding of the nature of the universe and its workings. The list is counterbalanced later in the quotation by another list, in this case a string of negatives: 'οὔτε . . . οὔτε . . . οὐδὲν, οὔτ' . . . οὐδενὸς . . . οὐ' 'not . . . nor . . . no, not . . . no . . . not'. The phrasing here conveys a call-and-response pattern, with the author then using the term 'opposite' to refer to their errors in treatment 'οὓς ἐχρῆν τἀντία τούτοισι ποιεῖν' 'They should have treated [these diseases] in the opposite way.' (*On the Sacred Disease*, 1.12). As in *On Ancient Medicine*, we find the agonistic context reflected in the phrasing of the treatise.

In the opening of this treatise, then, oppositional pairs are used in a limited but poignant way at the site of complex and subtle distinctions between the author's position and that of his opponents, and to emphasise his direct contradiction of his opponents' views.

(d) On the Art

The beginning of *On the Art* does not contain dense use of oppositional statements, unlike the opening of *On Breaths* or *On Ancient Medicine*. However, the first four sections of the treatise can be read as preliminary, leading up to a declaration of the subject of the treatise in Section 5. I will first briefly summarise the contents of the opening sections of the treatise, before going on to examine the use of oppositional pairs in the fifth section in more detail.

In Section 1 of *On the Art*, the author makes a powerful attack on those he claims make an art out of vilifying the arts. The author asserts in defence of the art that to discover what was unknown before is progress; he claims that this is the ambition and task of intelligence and notes that his treatise 'ἐναντιώσεται' 'will oppose' (1.2) attacks on the existence of the art of medicine. In Section 2, the author claims that it is absurd to think of something that plainly exists as non-existent. The author then asserts that he believes that the names of arts (including the art of medicine) have been attributed to them because they exist: their names indicate their existence, or real essence. He notes that it is also absurd, however, to think that real essence springs from names. In Section 3, the author states that he will discuss the art of medicine and offers a general definition of the art of medicine – 'τὸ δὴ πάμπαν ἀπαλλάσειν τῶν νοσεόντων τοὺς καμάτους καὶ τῶν νοσημάτων τὰς σφοδρότητας ἀμβλύειν, καὶ τὸ μὴ ἐγχειρεῖν τοῖσι κεκρατημένοισιν ὑπὸ τῶν νοσημάτων' 'to do away with the sufferings of the sick, to lessen the violence of their diseases, and to refuse to treat those who are overmastered by their diseases' (3.2). In Section 4, the author discusses the role of luck in recovery from illness and again counters the charge that the art of medicine does not exist.

Section 5 of the treatise, then, marks the beginning of the author's positive account of the art of medicine, in which he seeks to buttress his claims with arguments and 'τεκμήριον' 'proof' (5.3). In this section, we find the accumulation of pairs of opposing statements used as a kind of security for the point being made. The use of oppositional pairs in this section also echoes the agonistic context which is referred to in the previous four sections. The oppositions establish the moral authority of the speaker and dramatise and polarise the distinction between different physicians, so they have a sociological frame of reference similar to those used in the opening of *On Breaths*, and *On Ancient Medicine*. The oppositional pairs are as follows (see Tables 5.3 and 5.4 below).

The central oppositional pair – art (τέχνη) and luck (τύχη) – dominates the author's argument regarding the existence of the art of medicine in Sections 4 to 5. The author examines the case for the existence of the art of medicine and counter claims that the art of medicine is a figment of the imagination. Proof that the art exists lies, ultimately, in the claim that 'Πολλὴ γὰρ ἀνάγκη καὶ τοὺς μὴ χρεωμένους ἰητροῖσι, νοσήσαντας δὲ καὶ ὑγιασθέντας, εἰδέναι ὅτι ἢ δρῶντές τι ἢ μὴ δρῶντες ὑγιάνθησαν' 'Necessarily, those who did not consult a doctor but recovered after falling sick must know that they recovered by doing or not doing something.' (5.4) This claim is supported by a set of oppositions that echo and reinforce the 'doing-not doing' antithesis and refers to the way that medicine operates: by creating balance in the body through managing oppositions. By association, the method of countering extremes to produce a balance in the body relates to the weighing up of opposite arguments to ascertain the truth the preceding part of Sections 4 and 5.

In a further set of oppositions, the author claims that the presence of both elements of the oppositional pairs demonstrate the existence of the art of medicine: in other words, the fact that there exists a boundary between what is correct and incorrect, for example, denotes that there is an area of expertise in existence.

The second set of oppositional pairs builds upon the preceding sets, because the accumulation of oppositional pairs on each point helps build a sense of inevitability and plausibility to the claim that is being made. For want of any other way to demonstrate the existence of the art of medicine, the author uses association between oppositional pairs to show his command over medical

Table 5.3 Oppositions relating to proof of the existence of the art of medicine in *On the Art* 5.4[7]

fasting	feeding
thirst	drinking
not washing	washing
rest	exercise
being asleep	being awake

Table 5.4 Oppositions relating to the existence of the art of medicine in *On the Art* 5.5–6[8]

benefit	harm
praise	blame
correct	incorrect

matters by indicating his understanding of the underlying pattern. This underlying pattern also helps to secure his point, that expertise in this area must exist.

By examining the use of oppositions indicated in the tables above in context, we can understand more clearly how, in this section, the author suggests a process by which medical reasoning, which itself relies on a notion of opposition, occurs.

Section 5 refers to the use of arguments and counter arguments in the first line of the section: 'Ἐρεῖ δὴ ὁ τἀναντία λέγων ὅτι πολλοὶ ἤδη καὶ οὐ χρησάμενοι ἰητρῷ νοσέοντες ὑγιάσθησαν· καὶ ἐγὼ τῷ λόγῳ οὐκ ἀπιστέω.' 'Now the person who makes the opposite argument will say that many who were sick have recovered even without consulting a physician, and I do not doubt the claim' (5.1); this is followed by the author claiming that it is possible for lay people to chance upon medicine, though they will not know the difference between 'ὅ το ὀρθὸν ἐν αὐτῇ ἔνι ἢ ὅ τι μὴ ὀρθόν' 'what is correct in it and what is not' (5.2). Here, the author refers to arguments and counter-arguments for luck in recovery. He notes that the sick may recover without a physician, but uses another opposition to undermine the claim that this is purely by chance: the lay person will simply not realise what is correct method and what is not. The first opposition – between luck and the art of medicine – is undermined by another – between correct and incorrect method – by which the author lays claim to greater understanding.

In the following sentence, the author claims that he has 'τέκμήριον μέγα τῇ οὐσίῃ τῆς τέχνης ὅτι ἐοῦσά τέ ἐστι καὶ μεγάλη' 'powerful evidence of medicine's being – evidence that it both is and is powerful' (5.3). The evidence consists of a series of oppositional pairs, the first being included in the statement 'Πολλὴ γὰρ ἀνάγκη καὶ τοὺς μὴ χρεωμένους ἰητροῖσι, νοσήσαντας δὲ καὶ ὑγιασθέντας εἰδέναι, ὅτι ἢ δρῶντές τι ἢ μὴ δρῶντες ὑγιάνθησαν' 'Necessarily those who did not consult a doctor but recovered after falling sick must know that they recovered by doing or not doing something.' (5.4). The oppositional pair in this sentence – 'doing or not doing something' – is then echoed in a series of further oppositional pairs in the following sentence:

ἢ γὰρ ἀσιτίη, ἢ πολυφαγίη, ἢ ποτῷ πλέονι, ἢ δίψῃ, ἢ λουτροῖσιν ἢ ἀλουσίῃ ἢ πόνοισιν ἢ ἡσυχίῃ, ἢ ὕπνοισιν ἢ ἀγρυπνίῃ, ἢ τῇ ἀπάντων τούτων ταραχῇ χρεώμενοι ὑγιάνθησαν.

For it was by fasting or by overeating, by drinking much fluid or by abstaining from it, by bathing or by not bathing, by vigorous exercise or by rest, by sleep or wakefulness, or by using some combination of these that they recovered.

(5.4)

In this way, the 'powerful evidence' consists of the fact that patients recover through a range of binary options, the accumulation of which is a kind of catalogue of behaviours that point in the direction of a systematised body of knowledge. The form of the sentence here then suggests the existence of a systematised body of knowledge.

The author continues noting *how* learning can come about from experience:

Καὶ τῷ ὠφελῆσθαι πολλὴ ἀνάγκη αὐτούς ἐστιν ἐγνωκέναι ὅ τι ἦν τὸ ὠφελῆσαν, καὶ εἴ τι γ᾽ἐβλάβησαν, τῷ βλαβῆναι, ὅ τι ἦν τι τὸ βλάψαν. Τὰ γὰρ τῷ ὠφελῆσθαι καὶ τὰ τῷ βεβλάφθαι ὡρισμένα, οὐ πᾶς ἱκανὸς γνῶναι· Εἰ τοίνυν ἐπιστήσεται ἢ ἐπαινεῖν ἢ ψέγειν ὁ νοσήσας τῶν διαιτημάτων τι οἷσιν ὑγιάνθη, πάντα ταῦτα τῆς ἰητρικῆς ἐστι.

And they must through this have learnt by having benefited, what it was that benefited them, just as when they were harmed they must have learnt, by being harmed, what it was that harmed them. For it is not everybody who is capable of discerning things distinguished by benefit and things distinguished by harm. If therefore the patient knows how to praise or to blame what composed the regimen under which he or she recovered, all these things belong to the art of medicine.

(5.5)

The extract here hints at the processes by which understanding can come about, through a series of polarised issues. The focus on the ability to praise or blame implies that this treatise too – the defence of the art – is included within the notion of an art of medicine.

Finally, the author states:

Καίτοι ὅπου τό τε ὀρθὸν καὶ τὸ μὴ ὀρθὸν ὅρον ἔχει ἑκάστερον, πῶς τοῦτο οὐκ ἂν τέχνη εἴη; Τοῦτο γὰρ ἔγωγέ φημι ατεχνίην εἶναι ὅπου μήτε ὀρθὸν ἔνι μηδὲν μήτε οὐκ ὀρθόν· ὅπου δὲ τούτων ἔνεστιν ἑκάστερον, οὐκέτι ἂν τοῦτο ἔργον ἀτεχνίης εἴη.

Now where correctness and incorrectness each have a defined limit, surely there must be an art. For absence of art I take to be absence of correctness and of incorrectness; but where both are present art cannot be absent.

(5.6)

The existence of opposite categories is stated here to be evidence of the existence of art; this is ironically further supported by another antithetical contrast, between the presence of art and its absence. The entanglement of oppositional statements here is therefore doing the work of conveying secure evidence to the audience: as in all the examples above, interconnected oppositional pairs are being deployed by the author as firm evidence of his claim that the art of medicine exists to convey the soundness of his message and to articulate the processes through which medical learning occurs.

(e) On the Nature of Human Beings

There are some thematic oppositions in play throughout the first and second sections of *On the Nature of Human Beings*, in which the author counters the claims of his opponents that the human body is composed of only one element. These oppositions associate with one another to build up a complex argument against the author's opponents.

The oppositional pairs are follows: between the human being as formed of a single element and as formed of many; between the author's views as singular and true and those of his interlocutors all the same and flawed; and between rhetorical games and knowledge grounded in experience. These examples of opposition are less pronounced and used more subtly than in *On Breaths* or *On Ancient Medicine*, or Section 5 of *On the Art*, yet their presence nevertheless suggests adherence to a model opening of an oratorical treatise which is characterised by polar positioning between the speaker and his opponents.

The author shows through an interweaving of different oppositional points that, despite claims to the contrary, he is just as involved in the use of persuasive techniques as those he seeks to expose.

ἐμοὶ δὲ οὐδέν τι δοκεῖ ταῦτα οὕτως ἔχειν· οἱ μὲν οὖν πλεῖστοι τοιαῦτά τινα ἢ ὅτι ἐγγυτατα τούτων ἀποφαίνονται. ἐγὼ δέ φημι, εἰ ἓν ἦν ὤνθρωπος, οὐδέποτ' ἂν ἤλγει· οὐδὲ γὰρ ἂν ἦν ὑπ' ὅτευ ἀλγήσειεν ἓν ἐόν· εἰ δ' οὖν καὶ ἀλγήσειεν, ἀνάγκη καὶ τὸ ἰώμενον ἓν εἶναι· νῦν δὲ πολλά· πολλὰ γάρ ἐστιν ἐν τῷ σώματι ἐνεόντα, ἅ, ὅταν ὑπ'ἀλλήλων παρὰ φύσιν θερμαίνεταί τε καὶ ψύχηται, καὶ ξηραίνηται καὶ ὑγραίνηται, νούσους τίκτει· ὥστε πολλαὶ μὲν ἰδέαι τῶν νοσημάτων, πολλὴ δὲ ἡ ἴησίς ἐστιν. ἀξιῶ δ'ἐγὼ τὸν φάσκοντα αἷμα μοῦνον εἶναι τὸν ἄνθρωπον, καὶ ἄλλο μηδέν, δεικνύειν αὐτὸ[ν] μήτε μεταλλάσσον[τα] τὴν ἰδέην μηδὲ γίνομενον παντοῖον, ἀλλ' ἢ ὥρην τινὰ τοῦ ἐνιαυτοῦ ἢ τῆς ἡλικίης τῆς τοῦ ἀνθρώπου, ἐν ᾗ αἷμα ἐνεὸν φαίνεται μοῦνον ἐν τῷ ἀνθρώπῳ . . .

But, in my opinion, this is not the case. Most people put forward similar or closely related theories, but I believe that were the human being a unity he would not feel pain. Let's suppose that a human being suffered; necessarily, the cure would also be singular but in fact there exist many cures. There exist many elements in the body that by a reciprocal action can heat up, cool down, dry out or moisten contrary to nature and in this way produce disease. So there are many forms of disease and many modes of treatment. I think that the person who claims that the human being is just blood, and nothing else, should demonstrate that this element does not change form nor undergo multiple modifications, and that there exists a period either of the year or in the life of a human during which the blood is manifestly the single element of the human.

(2.3–2.4)

The main contrast in this extract is between the claims made by the author's opponents which state that the human body is formed of one element and the evidence from the human body which the author claims indicates diversity of elements. The author argues that most people propose ('ἀποφαίνονται') theories that the human being is a unity, but contends that if it were a unity it would not feel pain. At the same time, he is claiming that the *theories* of his opponents are the same or nearly so. He thus associates his own position with that of the body – the human body shows diverse elements and the author also claims that diverse elements exist in the body. In this way, he attacks his opponents, who claim that the human body is formed of a single element. Furthermore, he undermines the range of different claims made by his opponents – that the body is composed of one element or another – by stating that they are all in fact the same in the sense that no matter which element is referred to, they all claim that the human body is composed of only one element.

In other words, the author argues that (1) the theory of a single element which is the material of all human beings is wrong because the human being is composed of many different elements; (2) that the *theorists* who claim that the human being is made of a single element all say the same thing and are all wrong because just as the human being is composed of many different elements, so there are many different cures for its ailments. The author displaces the theory that the human body is composed of one element onto his opponents: they all say the same thing, he claims, whereas the human body shows diversity.

The human body, then, is a kind of third character in this account, additional to the speaker and the opponents. The human body is characterised as complex because of its diversity of aspects and functions. Similarly, the author's views are presented as complex because they encompass a wide range of topics and theories. The author's opponents' views of the body, on the other hand, are naïve: although they appear to be different, they are all the same; similarly, the opponents' views of the human body are wrong because they fail to acknowledge the different elements present in the human body. The opponents' attempts at understanding the body aim at diversity yet this diversity is revealed by the author of this treatise to mask similarity and therefore also to mask simple-mindedness or shallow-mindedness.

*

To draw some conclusions from this section of the chapter, we have seen how antitheses play a range of persuasive functions in the openings of the five Hippocratic oratorical treatises examined.

In *On Breaths* oppositions serve as follows: to attract attention, to build drama, to emphasise and/or establish social hierarchy, to make an associative link between moral rectitude and bodily health, to support by emphasis and repetition the key theory that opposites are cures for opposites and that, by implication, the use of oppositional pairs as part of the persuasive strategy has a corrective or even therapeutic value.

In *On Ancient Medicine*, the use of oppositions in the opening of the treatise is somewhat more complex than in *On Breaths*, as a range of other persuasive features are also employed alongside binary pairs, including complementary pairs and listing. As with *On Breaths*, there is some associative value between binary pairs, for example between truth and falsehood and the old medical methods and medical innovations: there is, then a strong moral element to the oppositions in this case, and moralising vocabulary is employed to further strengthen their persuasive force. Overall, the opening shows anxiety about the absence of any standard by which to measure the truth of one theory against another; and the range of persuasive strategies in place, including the use of oppositional pairs, is intended to undermine the singularity and simplicity of the theories of the monists by conveying complexity.

In *On the Sacred Disease* we have seen how, at the start of the treatise, oppositional pairs are used in a limited but poignant way at the site of complex and subtle distinctions between the author's position and that of his opponents.

In *On the Art*, we find dense use of oppositional statements in Section 5 of the treatise, which is where the author announces that he is beginning fully to discuss his topic proper – the art of medicine as opposed to *techne* in general. The oppositional pairs in this section serve to establish the security of the point being made through their accumulation; echo the agonistic context in which the treatise is delivered; help to establish the moral and sociological authority of the speaker; and convey a sense of a systematised body of knowledge. We also find an entanglement of oppositional statements towards the end of the section which serve to assert the author's authority both through the complexity of their entangled form, which implies the complexity of the author's knowledge and understanding, and through the main content of the oppositions, which is polarisation of the existence and inexistence of the art of medicine.

In *On the Nature of Human Beings*, we find oppositional pairs used less prominently, though perhaps more subtly and complexly, than in other 'oral' Hippocratic treatises examined here; their presence nevertheless suggests that the author is adhering to a model opening of a treatise at some level. In the second section of the treatise, we find the author using a polar opposition between sameness and difference to serve as a psychological rebuttal of his opponents' views in a complex set of oppositional pairs which serve to undermine his opponents as naïve and erroneous in their views through a complex entanglement of associations between sameness and difference in the composition of the body and in the theoretical position of the author and his opponents.

Associative oppositions as formulae and implied moralising in *On Ancient Medicine*

In the following parts of this chapter, I go on to discuss the association between oppositions in *On Ancient Medicine* and *On the Sacred Disease* in more detail. In the case of *On Ancient Medicine*, there is evidence for formulaic use of oppositions throughout the treatise which serve to build up a set of moral associations that lurk in the hinterland to the main accounts presented. In the case of *On the Sacred Disease*, I consider two recent investigations into the use of rhetoric in this treatise and the issue of how far the author can be understood to hold a coherent theological outlook. In this discussion, I will suggest that associative persuasive patterning based on oppositional structures can help us to better understand the author's meaning and theological outlook.

As well as being used for the purposes outlined above to herald the beginning of a treatise, we also find examples of oppositions used in *On Ancient Medicine* more elaborately and extensively than in *On Breaths*, *On the Art* or *On the Nature of Human Beings*, which associate with one another and serve to build a network of implied moral messages. Because of the degree of elaboration of their use in *On Ancient Medicine*, this treatise deserves further attention on this topic.

In Section 3 of *On Ancient Medicine*, the author gives an account of medicine's discovery, with its origins in the recognition that the same foods, drinks and regimen are not suitable for both healthy and sick people. This in turn is related to the way in which the diet of human beings became distinguished from the diet of other living beings in the distant past. The author places emphasis on a process of discovery elaborated over a long period of time during which human beings sought to alleviate their suffering, developing foodstuffs which were ever more apt for human consumption. The driving force for the development of medicine in this way, according to this author, is necessity, here given agency: 'αὐτὴ ἡ ἀνάγκη ἰητρικὴν ἐποίησε ζητηθῆναί τε καὶ εὑρεθῆναι ἀνθρώποισιν' 'But in fact necessity itself caused medicine to be sought for and discovered by human beings' (3.2, 2–4).

The section contains a series of binary oppositions: between the present day and the distant past; between animals and humans; between strong and weak foods and strong and weak human constitutions. The implied and more fundamental opposition is between the correct – natural – method of medical development and the incorrect method of the medical innovators who the author attacks in his treatise.

There is also an opposition between medicine as a heroic art and suffering and disease with which the section culminates: 'εὕρηται ἐπὶ τῇ τοῦ ἀνθρώπου ὑγιείῃ τε καὶ σωτηρίῃ καὶ τροφῇ, ἄλλαγμα κείνης τῆς διαίτης ἐξ ἧς οἱ πόνοι καὶ νοῦσοι καὶ θάνατοι ἐγίνοντο' 'it was discovered for the sake of the health, preservation, and nourishment of the human being, in place of that regimen which led to suffering, diseases and death' (3.6). Here, the opposition is underlined by a balance of three items in either half of the sentence ('ὑγιείῃ . . . τροφῇ . . . σωτηρίῃ' 'health . . . nourishment . . . preservation'; 'οἱ πόνοι . . . νοῦσοι . . . θάνατοι' 'suffering . . . diseases . . . death'). This latter opposition highlights the main thrust of the section overall that the only method by which medicine developed is the one being described, in that it seeks to convey the clear culmination of a natural progression: the correct method of pursuing the art of medicine is associated here with the development of human beings towards better health, nourishment and preservation. The phrase 'διὰ δὴ ταύτην τὴν χρείην καὶ οὗτοί μοι δοκέουσι ζητῆσαι τροφὴν ἁρμόζουσαν τῇ φύσει' 'It was on account of this need, I believe, that these people sought for nourishment suited to their constitution' (3.4) also further contributes to this sense of a natural path towards the discovery of medicine.

The moral point here, and the one that is produced from the association of different pairs of opposition, is that of the march of human progress away from the erroneous ways of the past and away from the absence of art or skill among animals. Nature and necessity are associated with one another, and by implication the author's opponents' methods are attacked as unnatural and unnecessary – though the author never explicitly states as much.[9]

As well as the associations between different oppositions implying a moral position, we also find examples in the treatise of the author describing in further detail the opposition between elements in the body, and how recovery from illness can be achieved by the balancing of one opposite with another. In doing so, the author makes reference both to physiological theory and to the persuasive, agonistic context of his theories: he speaks at the same time of medicine, the body and intellectual tribalism. To understand this point, we need to consider how different persuasive features of Section 19, towards the end of the treatise, operate persuasively in conjunction with one another.

The author begins Section 19 by giving an example of how changes to the quality of elements from pure to blended can lead to alleviation of symptoms. He describes a pattern of heat and inflammation being calmed by coction and thickening of fluxes, in this case of the covering of the eyeball. Similarly, fever accompanying fluxes in the throat is said to cool once the fluxes become thicker and more ripe and free of all acridness. Furthermore, the author states that these fluxes are the cause of the conditions (19.4).

In the second part of the section, the author moves on to generalise further, noting, with some exclamatory remarks, that so long as a humour is in an excited state and unblended, it causes suffering for the patient. The section ends with a general statement about the importance of mixing and with the general maxim that 'Πάντων δ᾽ἄριστα διάκειται ὤνθρωπος ὅταν πέσσηται καὶ ἐν ἡσυχίῃ ᾖ μηδεμίαν δύναμιν ἰδίην ἀποδεικνύμεθα· 'the human being is in the best possible condition whenever these [powers] are concocted or at rest, displaying no power of their own' (19.7).

The point that mixing of powers leads to the best possible condition for the human body stated above is explicitly linked by the author with earlier similar statements, to indicate his argument is built up cumulatively and consistently and to convey a breadth of coverage. The author begins this section by citing some examples of humoural theory continued from the previous section. The use of 'Ὅσα' adverbially meaning 'Next' (or 'just as') in at the beginning of 19.1 and 19.2 indicates that further examples of the theory already cited are being given and so the author seeks here to persuade through breadth of coverage. A rhetorical question is used to engage the audience and now to develop a call-and-response: Ὀδύναι δὲ καὶ καῦμα καὶ φλογμὸς ἔσχατος κατέχει μέχρι τινος; Μέχρι ἂν τὰ ῥεύματα πεφθῇ καὶ γένηται παχύτερα καὶ λήμη ἀπ᾽αὐτῶν ᾖ᾽ 'Pain and burning heat and extreme inflammation grip the patient, and for how long? Until the fluxes are concocted and become thicker and rheum is formed from them' (19.1). The pattern is by now obvious: pain, burning and inflammation are in place until elements are blended; this is also the overarching claim of this section.

Further examples and support for the claim through a range of evidence and emphatic statements making reference to necessary connections follow – for instance, the author reinforces the point that the elements themselves cause the ailment: 'Δεῖ δὲ δήπου ταῦτα αἴτια ἑκάστου ἡγεῖσθαι εἶναι, ὧν παρεόντων μὲν τοιουτότροπον ἀνάγκη γίνεσθαι . . . ' 'One should count as the cause of each complaint those things the presence of which of necessity produces a complaint of a certain kind' (19.3, 2–4) using the terms 'Δεῖ' 'One must' and 'ἀνάγκη' 'necessarily' to underline this. The main claim above – that in isolation elemental powers in the body cause distress and pain; blended they are unproblematic – is then repeated: 'ὅσον δ᾽ἂν χρόνον ταῦτα μετέωρα ᾖ καὶ ἄπεπτα καὶ ἄκρητα, μηχανὴ οὐδεμία οὔτε τῶν πόνων παύεσθαι οὔτε τῶν πυρετῶν.' 'But as long as these humors are in an excited state, unconcocted, and unblended, there is no way to be rid of either the pains or the fevers' (19.5).

The claim functions at different levels: it clearly refers to the mixing of elements in the human body; because of the persuasive context of the treatise, it also obliquely refers to the political tribalism the author attacks at the beginning of the treatise – with each opponent claiming that the human body consists of only one element. The innovators, then, this statement implies, are isolationists and like unconcocted, unblended elements in the body: as in the body disease is said to be aroused through separation and absence of harmony, so in the body politic of medical thinking.

The use of alpha privative to express this: 'ἄπεπτα καὶ ἄκρητα' 'uncon-cocted and unblended' helps to convey the unnaturalness of this situation, drawing on the associations between naturalness and the author's claims identified earlier in the treatise. The verb 'μετέωρα' 'in an excited state' from 'μετεωρίζω' which includes the meanings 'to raise to a height', 'to cause one to pant' and, more metaphorically 'to unsettle [the mind]' and 'to be anxious' covers both somatic and emotive fields of meaning, and helps this sentence to imply both mental and physical effects and thus the diseased body and the debate which is the context for this oratorical treatise.

The following sentence includes exclamatory remarks about the nature of diseases: 'οἷαι λύσσαι καὶ δήξιες σπλάγχνων καὶ θώρηκος καὶ ἀπορίη' 'what frenzy they suffer, what gnawings of the viscera and the chest, what distress!' (19.5). The terms 'λύσσαι . . . δήξιες . . . ἀπορίη' 'frenzy . . . gnawings . . . distress' can all be understood to relate to the physical body as well as to the mind ('δήξιες' can also refer to mental pangs and biting jokes).[10] The account here, then, turns to one of horror that overtakes the body and possibly also the mind, and again serves as a final underhand attack on the innovators whose theories are by implication obstructive in healing terrible disease and who may also be considered as a kind of social disease themselves. The use of 'κακοπαθεῖ' 'suffers' – a rather generic term for suffering – is the same term as used in Section 13, where the threat of 'πολλὰ καὶ δεινά' 'many terrible things' (13.1) is employed; here too, then, there seems to be a vague threat in play as to the dangers of unblended elements in the body, that is, the dangers of disruption of harmony.

In this way, the author draws on oppositional claims outlined earlier in the treatise, and builds up associations between physiological theory and persuasive context.

Overall, in *On Ancient Medicine*, cumulative sets of oppositions are being used to enforce a moral stance which the author uses to support his medical theory and help to associate his opponents with what is animalistic and 'unci-vilised', and his own theories with a greater degree of sophistication and civility. We find examples of oppositional statements resonating with one another throughout the treatise, forging suggestive connections between intellectual tribalism, medical theory and accounts of the function of the body, which culminate in the resonance between the notion of unconcocted elements in the body causing pain and illness, and warring intellectual medical factions. I now turn to an examination of the resonance between oppositional pairs in *On the Sacred Disease*, in light of recent scholarship on the rhetoric of this treatise.

Antithesis and explanation in *On the Sacred Disease*

Scholars have seen a tension between the opening of *On the Sacred Disease*, with its polemic against the magico-religious healers' understanding of seizure, and the positive account of the occurrence of seizure which occupies most of the remainder of the treatise.[11] This tension is one which impinges on the question of how we read the treatise: further examination of its use of antithesis and resonance between different parts of the treatise can go some way to explaining why flaws are observed in the linear logic of the author's explanation. I summarise briefly below the main points of interpretation relating to the question of the coherency of the theory in the treatise and then identify ways in which analysis of resonance between antithetical pairs can help to offer a fresh view on this problem.

In *The Art Is Long: On the Sacred Disease and the Scientific Tradition* (2002), Julie Laskaris notes, regarding the author's attack on magico-religious methods of treating seizure: 'Since the logic of [the author's] explanation of humoral balance does not demand it, why does the author employ a religious aetiology as well? . . . the author was compelled to formulate a religious framework for his mechanistic aetiology. To show that he could cure a sacred disease, he had to overcome the claims of his opponents . . . by showing that he was the superior in piety and in knowledge.' (2002: 123–124). She argues that the intellectual context of the treatise demanded that the author develop arguments not only to convince audiences regarding his notion of disease but also to counter the claims of magico-religious healers.

Laskaris comments on the use of the author's explanatory model of disease causation: 'Far from showing a willingness to question or reject a failed hypothesis or theoretical model, the author scrambles to produce *ad hoc* explanations, still keeping humoural imbalance as the ultimate cause, but relying upon a wide variety of ancillary causes and contingent factors as needed.' (2002: 77–78). Laskaris suggests here that the account of the development of the disease shows signs of being composed in a fashion which is not logically effective.

Philip van der Eijk, in his article 'The "Theology" of the Hippocratic Treatise *On the Sacred Disease*' (2005 [1990]) focuses on an inconsistency between the ideas concerning the divine expressed in the opening polemical section of the treatise and in the author's positive account of the disease. He notes that in scholarship on the divine character of the 'sacred' disease, there are basically 'two interpretations of the use of the words 'divine' (*theios*) and 'human' (*anthro͞pinos*)' (2005 [1990]: 48). Both interpretations are said to be based on the following passages: 1, 2; 2, 1–3; 18, 1–2 (=*On the Sacred Disease*, 1.1; 2.1; 18.1).

The first interpretation is that 'a disease is divine in virtue of being caused by factors . . . which are themselves divine' (2005 [1990]: 49). This interpretation rests mainly on the remark 'Ταῦτα δ'ἐστὶ θεῖα' 'these things are divine' (*On the Sacred Disease* 18.1) where '"these things" is taken as a reference to the "causes" (προφάσιες) mentioned in the previous sentence, "the things that come and go away etc." (τῶν προσιόντων καὶ ἀπιόντων κτλ.)' (2005 [1990]: 51).

The second interpretation is that 'the disease is divine in virtue of having a *phusis*, a 'nature' ([that is,] a regular pattern of origin and growth).' (2005 [1990]: 57). This interpretation is based principally on two key points in the treatise. The first point in the text is 'the mention of *phusis* in 1.2 and 2.1–2 [=*On the Sacred Disease* 1.1 and 2.1] in the immediate context of the claim that epilepsy is not more divine than other diseases'. The second point in the text is the phrase at 18.2 [=18.1] '"and each of them has a nature and a power of its own, and none is hopeless or impossible to deal with" (φύσιν δὲ ἕκαστον . . . οὐδ'ἀμήχανον)' which is read 'as providing the explanation of [the phrase] "all are divine and all are human" (πάντα θεῖα καὶ πάντα ἀνθρώπινα)' (2005 [1990]: 57).

Van der Eijk argues that neither interpretation is entirely convincing, but that the second involves fewer problems and is therefore preferable to the first (2005 [1990]: 60). He then goes on to focus on the limitations inherent in the extrapolation of the author's theology based on either of these interpretations or on a combination of both.

Van der Eijk notes that there are 'several implicit presuppositions [in the polemical opening of the treatise] which do not make sense within . . . a naturalistic conception of the divine.' (2005 [1990]: 60). He makes reference to the 'accusations of impiety (*asebeia*) and atheism (*atheos*) which begin in 1.28 [=1.4] . . . and which are continued in 1.39ff. [=1.5f.]' (2005 [1990]: 62). In particular, he notes that the author appears to have 'an explicit opinion on what is pious and what is not' (2005 [1990]: 63). Van der Eijk then refers to 1.44–6 [=1.13] (in which the author comments on the role of gods in purifying humans) as key to a search for the author's religious convictions. He interprets this passage as meaning that 'the writer believes in the reality of divine purification' and 'in gods who grant men purification of their moral transgressions and who are to be worshipped in temples by means of prayer and sacrifice' (2005 [1990]: 66–67). He concludes that 'If "the divine" mentioned in 1.45 [=1.13] is to be identified with the divine Nature or natural laws, it cannot be seen how this moral purification should be conceived within such a theology' (2005 [1990]: 67).

Overall, van der Eijk argues that the author is attempting to demarcate the boundaries between medicine and religion, but that there remains a tension between 'the author's belief in gods who cleanse men from their moral transgressions and his statements about the divine character of the disease.' (2005 [1990]: 69).

Van der Eijk concludes:

> The writer believes in gods who grant men purification of their trans-
> gressions and who are to be worshipped in temples by means of prayer
> and sacrifice. The text is silent on the author's conception of the nature
> of these gods, but there is, at least, no textual evidence that he rejected
> the notion of 'personal' or even 'anthropomorphic' gods. He has explicit
> opinions on how (and in what circumstances) these gods should be
> approached, and he definitely thinks it blasphemous to hold that these
> beings send diseases to men as pollutions. Diseases are not the effects of
> divine dispensation; nevertheless they have a divine aspect in that they
> show a constant and regular pattern of origin and development. How this
> 'being divine' is related to 'the divine' (or, the gods) which cleanses men
> from moral transgressions is not explained.
>
> (2005 [1990]: 70–71)

The connection between the notion that diseases 'are divine' and the author's
references to 'the divine' remains unresolved in this analysis and the 'theology' of the author, while detailed conjectures can be made and can establish the degree to which the Hippocratic author has a consistent set of ideas,
remains problematic.

Both van der Eijk and Laskaris refer, as a base for their analyses, to passages near the beginning and end of the treatise that establish the overall
framework and scope of the author's discussion. If, however, we look at these
passages with respect to attention to resonance of antithesis, a kind of coherence and continuity come into view that Laskaris' and van der Eijk's analyses
do not acknowledge. Let us first examine two passages near the beginning of
the treatise:

Περὶ τῆς ἱερῆς νούσου καλεομένης ὧδε ἔχει· οὐδέν τί μοι δοκεῖ τῶν
ἄλλων θειοτέρη εἶναι νούσων οὐδὲ ἱερωτέρη, ἀλλὰ φύσιν μὲν ἔχει καὶ
τὰ λοιπὰ νοσήματα ὅθεν γίνεται . . .

This is how things are with the so-called sacred disease. It is not, in my
opinion, any more divine or more sacred than other diseases, but has a
natural cause, and its supposed divine origin is due to people's inexperience, and to their wonder at its peculiar character . . .

(1.1)

Τὸ δὲ νόσημα τοῦτο οὐδέν τί μοι δοκεῖ θειότερον εἶναι τῶν λοιπῶν,
ἀλλὰ φύσιν μὲν ἔχειν καὶ τἆλλα νοσήματα ὅθεν ἕκαστα γίνεται, φύσιν
δὲ τοῦτο καὶ πρόφασιν, καὶ ἀπὸ ταὐτοῦ θεῖον γίνεσθαι ἀφ᾽ ὅτευ καὶ

τἆλλα πάντα, καὶ ἰητὸν εἶναι καὶ οὐδὲν ἧσσον ἑτέρων ὅ τι ἂν μὴ ἤδη ὑπὸ χρόνου πολλοῦ καταβεβιασμένον ἢ ὥστε ἤδη ἰσχυρότερον εἶναι τῶν φαρμάκων τῶν προσφερομένων.[12]

But this disease is in my opinion no more divine than any other; but just like other diseases which have a natural cause from which it is arises, this disease also has a natural cause; it is divine for the same reason as all the other diseases; it is also curable, no less than other illness, unless by long lapse of time it be so ingrained as to be more powerful than the remedies that are applied.

(2.1)

Both passages propose a generalisation about the 'sacred' disease. The first extract includes the phrase 'καὶ τὰ λοιπὰ νοσήματα' 'than other diseases', a tag used frequently throughout the treatise to connect individual phenomena with general phenomena and to enhance the breadth of coverage of the statement. The second extract contains two such tags 'καὶ τἆλλα νοσήματα' 'as other diseases' and 'καὶ τἆλλα πάντα' 'as all other diseases', the latter containing the term 'πάντα' 'all', which emphasises the status of the remark as universally applicable.

In these passages, the author attempts to communicate the idea that the 'sacred' disease is like all other diseases because it has a nature and a cause. The author wishes here to fit the 'sacred' disease into a neat generalisation about all diseases, a generalisation that is underscored by key tags that recur throughout the treatise.

Let us next turn to an extract from towards the end of the treatise:

Αὕτη δὲ ἡ νοῦσος ἡ ἱερὴ καλεομένη ἐκ τῶν αὐτῶν προφασίων γίνεται ἀφ᾽ ὧν καὶ αἱ λοιπαί, ἀπὸ τῶν προσιόντων καὶ ἀπιόντων, καὶ ψύχεος καὶ ἡλίου καὶ πνευμάτων μεταβαλλομένων τε καὶ οὐδέποτε ἀτρεμιζόντων. Ταῦτα δ᾽ ἐστὶ θεῖα ὥστε μηδὲν ἀποκρίνοντα τὸ νόσημα θειότερον τῶν λοιπῶν νομίζειν, ἀλλὰ πάντα θεῖα καὶ πάντα ἀνθρώπινα· φύσιν δὲ ἕκαστον ἔχει καὶ δύναμιν ἐφ᾽ ἑωυτοῦ, καὶ οὐδὲν ἄπορόν ἐστιν οὐδ᾽ ἀμήχανον·

This disease called sacred comes from the same causes as others, from the things that come to and go from the body, and from cold and sun and from the winds that change and are never motionless. These things are divine, so that there is no need to put this disease in a special class and to consider it more divine than others; they are all divine and all human. Each has a nature and power of its own and none is hopeless or incapable of treatment.

(18.1)

The phrases 'τῶν προσιόντων καὶ ἀπιόντων' 'things that come to and go away from [the body]' and 'ψύχεος καὶ ἡλίου' 'cold and sun' are polarities. One set of polar opposites recalls another set in the treatises (for example between phlegmatic and bilious, between clean and unclean and between north and south winds). The use of polarities here is suggestive, rather than fully explicative of the kinds of things that influence the development of the disease.

The author introduces polarities here as a reminder of the key character of his account. These phrases advertise the regularity and intelligibility of the causes of the disease but are not a list of specific items that are the 'same causes' as other diseases. Furthermore, they can be described as an example of *epangelma* but again it does not follow that the author now refers to his aim at the outset of the treatise to show that a complete and consistent analysis has been carried out, as would be expected from a treatise following a linear explanation.

In the passages from the beginning of the treatise quoted above, we also find a polarity between the 'sacred' disease which is the same as all the other diseases and the 'sacred' disease which is different from all other diseases: the author presents no middle ground between what is and what is not the case in these passages as the basis for his general claim that only one of these polar opposites is valid. The polarities noted at the end of the treatise loosely recall this first polarity, though of course the context of each polarity (e.g. as an aspect of argumentation, or as an aspect of the character of human constitution or climate) is very different.

Furthermore, the expression 'Ταῦτα δ' ἐστὶ θεῖα' 'these things are divine' in the second sentence of this passage is followed by the expression 'πάντα θεῖα καὶ πάντα ἀνθρώπινα' 'all things are divine and all things are human'. The author is attempting here to collapse the distinction between 'divine' and 'human' here. In the first sentence, the author's claim that 'these things are divine' may refer to the 'causes' understood as 'things that come and go' and - or that is to say - 'cold and sun and winds' as van der Eijk notes (2005 [1990]: 51 and 53). The emphasis in the sentence is on the idea of 'μηδὲν αποκρίνοντα' 'not separating'. The author does, from a logical point of view, contradict himself here (he states first that these things are divine, then that all things are human and divine). However, the accumulation of generalisations chimes with accumulations of generalisations elsewhere in the treatise.

The slight ambiguity of reference here (it is not absolutely clear what the word 'ταῦτα' 'these things' refers to, as just noted above) may remind us of the ambiguity of reference which, as we saw in previous chapters, is an important and influential feature of Heraclitus' writing.[13] The use of opposition is also in part, it seems, intentionally confusing: form is being sacrificed to content here. In other words, the author is not specific about what exactly is divine or what exactly is natural, nor about his explicit understanding of these terms; but the form of the text at this point is consistent with patterns we have seen throughout the treatise which aim to communicate a *sense* of coherence and authoritative understanding and reflects the prose of earlier writers such as Heraclitus. Furthermore, the opposition that is being introduced here between the one and the many, between what is or is not specific to the individual and what is general, also reminds us of the same opposition in Heraclitus.[14]

These lines could be viewed as developing those at the beginning of the treatise in the following way: whereas before it was said that the 'sacred' disease is not different to any other, here it is said that all diseases are the same in one respect and all different in another, thus offering an even more widely applicable generalisation. Throughout the course of his treatise, the author builds one generalisation on another and then culminates in offering an even broader generalisation at the end.

Let us turn to one final extract from the treatise:

Οὐ μέντοι ἔγωγε ἀξιῶ ὑπὸ θεοῦ ἀνθρώπου σῶμα μιαίνεσθαι, τὸ ἐπικηρότατον ὑπὸ τοῦ ἀγνοτάτου· ἀλλὰ κἢν τυγχάνῃ ὑφ᾽ ἑτέρου μεμιασμένον ἤ τι πεπονθός, ὑπὸ τοῦ θεοῦ καθαίρεσθαι ἂν αὐτὸ καὶ ἁγνίζεσθαι μᾶλλον ἢ μιαίνεσθαι. Τὰ γοῦν μέγιστα τῶν ἁμαρτημάτων καὶ ἀνοσιώτατα τὸ θεῖόν ἐστι τὸ καθαῖρον καὶ ἁγνίζον καὶ ῥύμμα γινόμενον ἡμῖν· αὐτοί τε ὅρούς τοῖσι θεοῖσι τῶν ἱρῶν καὶ τῶν τεμενέων ἀποδείκνυμεν, ὡς ἂν μηδεὶς ὑπερβαίνῃ ἢν μὴ ἁγνεύῃ, εἰσιόντες τε περιρραινόμεθα οὐχ ὡς μιαινόμενοι, ἀλλ᾽ εἴ τι καὶ πρότερον ἔχομεν μύσος, τοῦτο ἀφαγνιούμενοι. Καὶ περὶ μὲν τῶν καθαρμῶν οὕτω μοι δοκεῖ ἔχειν.

However, I hold that a man's body is not defiled by a god, the one being utterly corrupt, the other perfectly holy. Even should it have been defiled or in any way injured through some different agency, a god is more likely to purify and sanctify it than he is to cause defilement. At least it is godhead that purifies, sanctifies and cleanses us from the greatest and most impious of our sins; and we ourselves fix boundaries to the sanctuaries and precincts of the gods, so that nobody may cross them unless he be pure; and when we enter we sprinkle ourselves, not as defiling ourselves thereby, but to wash away any pollution we may have already contracted. This is my opinion about purifications.

(1.13)

Through the opposition 'most corruptible / most holy', the author here emphasises the distinction between the divine and the holy. This opposition is rephrased in the next sentence that claims that the most impious transgressions are cleansed by the divine, with the superlatives 'greatest' and 'most impious' implying and emphasising the contrast with the purity of the divine. These distinctions are part of a general pattern of oppositions that runs through the treatise and which, as we have seen above, is collapsed at the end of the trea-tise in the phrase 'πάντα θεῖα καὶ πάντα ἀνθρώπινα' 'all things are divine and all human' (18.1). Furthermore, these polar oppositions, as well as the refer-ence to marking the boundaries of the sanctuaries, resonate with the ongoing themes of categorisation that run through the treatise that are most prominent in the author's discussion of the different constitutions of human beings and in his discussion of the expulsion of excess phlegm in the brain of the embryo.

The above comments do not serve to resolve the tension between the differ-ent conceptions of the divine in the polemical section of the treatise and in the positive account of disease causation that both van der Eijk and Laskaris con-sider exists from the point of view of defining the author's theology. However, these comments do indicate that a consistency between the different parts of the treatise can still be found, on a level that might be dismissed as stylistic, but is in fact central to both the author's conception of his subject matter and his expressive resources.

In conclusion, we have seen in this chapter how oppositional pairs tend to feature at or near the opening of oratorical Hippocratic treatises and serve to establish a framework for the topic of each treatise as well as to echo, emphasise and articulate a response to the agonistic context for which they all appear to have been composed. We have also seen how chains of oppositional pairs tend to accumulate, forging underlying associations. This can serve to enhance the author's authoritative stance and the sense that there is a coherent line of thinking which is being explained. In more subtle and complex exam-ples, we find oppositional pairs relating to different contexts – physiology and intellectual tribalism in *On Ancient Medicine*, for instance – working in conjunction with one another to imply a moral attack on the opponents, and to help align the author's theories with perceived existing patterns in the body and so make them seem 'natural' or obvious.

We have also seen how in *On the Sacred Disease*, the resonance between oppositional pairs is an aspect of the author's explanatory framework, and that though associations between oppositions do not always yield consistent points of theory, their presence has an important persuasive value that is missed if we read the treatise only for its use of linear logical progression of thought. These points serve to support the argument developed throughout this book that Hippocratic oratorical treatises look back to earlier models of prose writ-ing as well as forward in terms of their experiment with form and innovations in theory.

Notes

1 For example, the treatise compares those living in cities exposed to hot winds and sheltered from the north winds in Section 3 with those living in cities exposed to cold winds and sheltered from the hot winds in Section 4. Likewise, the author

compares peoples of Europe with peoples of Asia in Section 12, noting that everything in Asia grows to far greater beauty and size, and in Section 12 and 14 that the inhabitants of Asia are milder and more gentle than their European counterparts.

2 'il consciente riuso del *polar thinking* può assumere nel *PM* la consistenza di un organon logica. Al di qua di strutture sillogistiche formali, il semplice andamento frastico giocato su coppie sinonimiche o antithetiche istituisce parallelismi e chiasmi, suggerendo per loro tramite mediate identificazioni . . .'
'Chiasmus' (literally 'crossing' from the Greek 'χίασμα') is the figure of speech in which two or more clauses are related to each other through a reversal of order of words or phrases.

3 See Clarke Kosak (2004) for further discussion of the representation of the physician as hero in *On Breaths* and other Hippocratic treatises.

4 'Εἰσί τινες τῶν τεχνέων αἳ τοῖσι μὲν κεκτημένοισίν εἰσιν ἐπίπονοι, τοῖσι δὲ χρεωμένοισιν ὀνήϊστοι, καὶ τοῖσι μὲν δημότησιν ξυνὸν ἀγαθόν, τοῖσι δὲ μεταχειριζομένοισί σφας λυπηραί. Τῶν δὲ δὴ τοιούτοων ἐστὶν τεχνέων καὶ ἥν οἱ Ἕλληνες καλέουσιν ἰητρικήν. ὁ μὲν γὰρ ἰητρὸς ὁρεῖ τε δεινά, θιγγάνει τε ἀηδέων, ἐπ᾽ ἀλλοτρίῃσί τε συμφορῇσιν ἰδίας καρποῦται λύπας· οἱ δὲ νοσέοντες ἀποτρέπονται διὰ τὴν τέχνην τῶν μεγίστων κακῶν, νούσων, λύπης, πόνων, θανάτου· πᾶσι γὰρ τούτοισιν ἄντικρυς ἰητρική. Ταύτης δὲ τῆς τέχνης τὰ μὲν φλαῦρα χαλεπὸν γνῶναι, τὰ δὲ σπουδαῖα ῥηΐδιον· καὶ τὰ μὲν φλαῦρα τοῖσιν ἰητροῖσι μούνοισιν ἔστιν εἰδέναι, καὶ οὐ τοῖσιν δημότησιν· οὐ γὰρ σώματος, ἀλλὰ γνώμης ἐστὶν ἔργα. Ὅσα μὲν γὰρ χειρουργῆσαι χρὴ συνεθισθῆναι δεῖ – τὸ γὰρ ἔθος τῇσι χερσὶ κάλλιστον διδασκαλεῖον –, περὶ δὲ τῶν ἀφανεστάτων καὶ χαλεπωτάτων νουσημάτων δόξῃ μᾶλλον ἢ τέχνη κρίνεται· διαφέρει δ᾽ἐν αὐτοῖσι πλεῖστον ἡ πείρα τῆς ἀπειρίης. . . . [1.5] Ὁ δὲ τοῦτ᾽ ἄριστα ποιέων ἄριστος ἰητρός, ὁ δὲ τούτου πλεῖστον ἀπολειφθεὶς πλεῖστον ἀπελείφθη τῆς τέχνης.'
'There are some arts which to those that possess them are painful, but to those that use them are helpful, a common good to laymen, but to those that practise them grievous. Of such arts there is one which the Greeks call medicine. For the physician sees terrible sights, touches unpleasant things, and the misfortunes of others bring a harvest of sorrows that are peculiarly his; but the sick by means of the art rid themselves of the worst of evils, disease, suffering, pain and death. For medicine proves for all these evils a manifest cure. And of this art, the bad aspects are difficult to understand while the good aspects are easier to comprehend; the bad aspects cannot be known except by physicians alone and not by laypeople; for they are matters of understanding, not of the body. For whenever surgical treatment is required, training by habituation is necessary – habit proves the best teacher of the hands –; but to judge of the most obscure and difficult diseases is more a matter of opinion than of art, and therein is revealed the greatest possible difference between experience and inexperience. . . . [1.5] He who performs these tasks is the best physician; he who is farthest removed from them is also farthest removed from the art' (*On Breaths*, 1.1–3; 1.5).

5 'Αὐτίκα γὰρ λιμὸς νοῦσός ἐστιν· ὅ γὰρ ἂν λυπῇ τὸν ἄνθρωπον, τοῦτο καλεῖται νοῦσος· Τί οὖν λιμοῦ φάρμακον; Ὅ παύει λιμόν· τοῦτο δ᾽ἐστὶ βρῶσις· τούτῳ ἄρα ἐκεῖνο ἰητέον. Αὖτις αὖ δίψαν ἔπαυσε πόσις· πάλιν αὖ πλησμονὴν ἰᾶται κένωσις· κένωσιν δὲ πλησμονή, πόνον δὲ ἀπονίη· ἀπονίην δὲ πόνος. Ἑνὶ δὲ συντόμῳ λόγῳ, τὰ ἐναντία τῶν ἐναντίων ἐστὶν ἰήματα· ἰητρικὴ γάρ ἐστιν ἀφαίρεσις καὶ πρόσθεσις, ἀφαίρεσις μὲν τῶν πλεοναζόντων, πρόσθεσις δὲ τῶν ἐλλειπόντων'
'For example, hunger is a disease, as everything is called a disease which makes a human being suffer. What then is the cure for hunger? Whatever suppresses

hunger. This is eating; so that by eating hunger must be cured. Another example: drink suppresses thirst; and again repletion cured by depletion, depletion by repletion, fatigue by rest. To sum up in a single sentence, opposites are cures for opposites. For medicine is subtraction and addition, subtraction of what is in excess, addition of what is lacking.' (*On Breaths*, 1.4–5).

6　For further discussion of blame and infertility in the Hippocratic Collection, see Fallas (2015: esp. 195–245) (Chapters 8–9). In examining cases where blame arises and its absence in relation to infertility, Fallas touches on the strong presence in the Collection of physicians' claims that will protect their reputations and interests, as well as on the presence of competing narratives regarding knowledge and experience, and the challenge to women's voices in particular.

7　'Πολλὴ γὰρ ἀνάγκη καὶ τοὺς μὴ χρωμένους ἰητροῖσι, νοσήσαντας δὲ καὶ ὑγιασθέντας, εἰδέναι, ὅτι ἢ δρῶντές τι ἢ μὴ δρῶντες ὑγιάσθησαν· ἢ γὰρ ἀσιτίη, ἢ πολυφαγίη, ἢ ποτῷ πλέονι, ἢ δίψῃ, ἢ λουτροῖσιν ἢ ἀλουσίη ἢ πόνοισιν ἢ ἡσυχίῃ, ἢ ὕπνοισιν ἢ ἀγρυπνίη, ἢ τῇ ἁπάντων τούτων ταραχῇ χρεώμενοι ὑγιάνθησαν.'

'Necessarily, those who did not consult a doctor but recovered after falling sick must know that they recovered by doing or not doing something. For it was by fasting or by overeating, by drinking much fluid or by abstaining from it, by bathing or by not bathing, by vigorous exercise or by rest, by sleep or wakefulness, or by using some combination of these that they recovered.'

(*On the Art*, 5.4)

8　'Καὶ τῷ ὠφελῆσθαι πολλὴ ἀνάγκη αὐτοὺς ἐστιν ἐγνωκέναι ὅ τι ἦν τὸ ὠφελῆσαν, καὶ εἴ τι γ᾽ ἐβλάβησαν, τῷ βλαβῆναι, ὅ τι ἦν τι τὸ βλάψαν. Τὰ γὰρ τῷ ὠφελῆσθαι καὶ τὰ τῷ βεβλάφθαι ὡρισμένα, οὐ πᾶς ἱκανὸς γνῶναι· Εἰ τοίνυν ἐπιστήσεται ἢ ἐπαινεῖν ἢ ψέγειν ὁ νοσήσας τῶν διαιτημάτων τι οἶσιν ὑγιάνθη, πάντα ταῦτα τῆς ἰητρικῆς ἐστι. Καί ἐστιν οὐδὲν ἧσσον τὰ ἁμαρτηθέντα τῶν ὠφελησάντων μαρτύρια τῇ τέχνῃ ἐς τὸ εἶναι. Τὰ μὲν γὰρ ὠφελήσαντα τῷ ὀρθῶς προσενεχθῆναι ὠφέλησε, τὰ δὲ βλάψαντα τῷ μηκέτι ὀρθῶς προσενεχθῆναι ἔβλαψε. Καίτοι ὅπου τό τε ὀρθὸν καὶ τὸ μὴ ὀρθὸν ὅρον ἔχει ἑκάστερον, πῶς τοῦτο οὐκ ἂν τέχνη εἴη; Τοῦτο γὰρ ἔγωγέ φημι ἀτεχνίην εἶναι ὅπου μήτε ὀρθὸν ἔνι μηδὲν μήτε οὐκ ὀρθόν.'

'And they must through this have learnt by having been benefited, what it was that benefited them, just as when they were harmed they must have learnt, by being harmed, what it was that harmed them. For it is not everybody who is capable of discerning things distinguished by benefit and things distinguished by harm. If therefore the patient knows how to praise or to blame what composed the regimen under which he or she recovered, all these things belong to the art of medicine. Again, mistakes, no less than benefits, witness to the existence of the art; for what benefited did so because correctly administered, and what harmed did so because incorrectly administered. Now where correctness and incorrectness each have a defined limit, surely there must be an art. For absence of art I take to be absence of correctness and of incorrectness' (*On the Art*, 5.5–6).

9　Similarly, in Section 8 of *On Ancient Medicine*, the author compares the consequences of making an error in the regimen of a sick person with a healthy person eating food suitable for an ox or a horse. The aim of the comparison is to illustrate that by trial and error, a suitable regimen for all kinds of conditions can be found; here too there is an underlying message which is hinted at: that health is associated with 'civilised' humanity and sickness or disease with what is 'uncivilised' or animalistic.

10　δῆξις, εως, ἡ, (δάκνω) 'bite', 'biting', Arist.HA623a1; δήξιες ϛπλάγχνων 'gnawings', Hp.VM19: metaph., of mental anguish, pangs, Zeno Stoic.1.51 (pl.),

Chrysipp.ib.3.119, Phld.D.3.Fr.22; also, 'biting jokes', Plu.Lyc.14. (Pantelia (2016) / *Thesaurus Linguae Graecae*).

11 For analysis of how closely the 'sacred' disease corresponds to modern understanding of epilepsy and seizure see Temkin (1971: 15–21).

12 The Greek text here differs somewhat from the text printed in Jones' 1998 [1923] edition, which reads: 'Τὸ δὲ νόσημα τοῦτο οὐδέν τί μοι δοκεῖ θειότερον εἶναι τῶν λοιπῶν, ἀλλὰ φύσιν ἔχει ἥν καὶ τὰ ἄλλα νοσήματα, καὶ πρόφασιν ὅθεν ἕκαστα γίνεται· καὶ ἰητον εἶναι, καὶ οὐδὲν ἧσσον ἑτέρων, ὅ τι ἂν μὴ ἤδη ὑπὸ χρόνου πολλοῦ καταβεβιασμένον ᾖ, ὥστε ἤδη ἰσχυρότερον εἶναι τῶν φαρμάκων τῶν προσφερομένων.'
    'But this disease is in my opinion no more divine that any other; it has the same nature as other diseases, and the cause that gives rise to individual diseases. It is also curable, no less than other illnesses, unless by long lapse of time it be so ingrained as to be more powerful than the remedies that are applied.' (Jones 1998 [1923]: 150–151).

13 See, for example, the ambiguous use of 'ὅδε', 'ἐκεῖνος' and 'οὗτος' in DK22B88 [Plutarch] *Consolation to Apollonius* 106e.

14 See e.g. DK22B114, Strobaeus 3.1.179.

References

Barton, J. (2005), 'Hippocratic Explanations' in van der Eijk, Ph. J. (ed.), *Hippocrates in Context: Papers Read at the XIth International Hippocrates Colloquium; (University of Newcastle upon Tyne, 27–31 August 2002)*. Leiden: Brill. 29–47.

Clarke Kosak, J. (2004), *Heroic Measures: Hippocratic Medicine in the Making of Euripidean Tragedy*. Leiden; Boston, MA: Brill.

van der Eijk, Ph. J. (2005), 'The "Theology" of the Hippocratic Treatise *On the Sacred Disease*' in van der Eijk, Ph. J. (ed.), *Medicine and Philosophy in Classical Antiquity. Doctors and Philosophers on Nature, Soul, Health and Disease*. Cambridge; New York: Cambridge University Press. 45–73 [first published in Apeiron 23 (1990), 87–119].

Fallas, R. M. (2015), *Infertility, Blame and Responsibility in the Hippocratic Corpus*. The Open University. PhD thesis.

Fantuzzi, M. (1983), 'Varianza e tenacia del *polar thinking* nel *De prisca medicina* pseudippocratico' in Lasserre, F. and Mudry, P. (eds.), *Formes de pensées dans la collection hippocratique: actes du IVe Colloque International Hippocratique (Lausanne, 21–26 septembre 1981)*. Genève: Librairie Droz. 233–248.

Hall, E. (1989), *Inventing the Barbarian: Greek Self-definition through Tragedy*. Oxford: Clarendon Press.

Jones, W. H. S. (ed. and trans.) (1998) [1923], *Hippocrates II*. Cambridge, MA; London, England: Harvard University Press.

Kahn, C. H. (1979), *The Art and Thought of Heraclitus: An Edition of the Fragments with Translation and Commentary*. Cambridge; New York: Cambridge University Press.

Laskaris, J. (2002), *The Art Is Long: On the Sacred Disease and the Scientific Tradition*. Leiden; Boston, MA: Brill.

Lloyd, G. E. R. (1966), *Polarity and Analogy: Two Types of Argumentation in Early Greek Thought*. Cambridge: Cambridge University Press.

Pantelia, M. C. (2016) (ed.) (accessed Dec. 10, 2016), *Thesaurus Linguae Graecae Digital Library*. Irvine: University of California. www.tlg.uci.edu.

Temkin, O. (1971), *The Falling Sickness: A History of Epilepsy from the Greeks to the Beginnings of Modern Neurology*. Baltimore, MD; London: Johns Hopkins University Press.

Conclusion

This book has set out to demonstrate, through an analysis of five Hippocratic treatises written with oral delivery in mind – *On Ancient Medicine* (*De vetere medicina*), *On the Art* (*De arte*), On *Breaths* (*De flatibus*), *On the Sacred Disease* (*De morbo sacro*), *On the Nature of Human Beings* (*De natura hominum*) – that Hippocratic expository prose represents evidence not only of major developments in medical understanding and philosophical debate about the nature of the human body and its ailments, but also of a significant contribution to the development of prose writing in ancient Greece.

By analysing the persuasive function of recurring patterns in language use in these treatises – such as antithesis and balancing effects in phrasing, repetitions and accumulations of words and phrases, tags, and use of rhyme and sound effects – we have seen how layers of meaning emerge which operate beyond the surface content of these texts and indicate the existence in the Hippocratic Collection of a variety of manners and modes of communication modelled on the work of early trailblazers in prose writing including Pre-Socratic and Sophistic writers and Herodotus.

We have also seen how scholarship on persuasive strategies and features of early Greek prose, including Hippocratic writing, has often tended to prioritise the linear logic of argument over analysis of implied meanings established through networks of associations and formulaic expression; the richness of Hippocratic expository prose has sometimes been overlooked and the extent to which it represents an attempt to establish a new medical *logos* or *logoi* – mixing persuasive and empirically argued elements – has been underestimated. This book has sought to complement existing studies on Hippocratic expository prose writing by shedding new light on the complexity of its poetics.

In Chapter 1, we saw how around ten to fifteen of the roughly seventy treatises of the Hippocratic Collection show a particularly close kinship with the more elaborate and ambitious prose writing and oratorical display texts of the period in which they were composed and so should be considered as significant evidence for the development of performance prose, alongside Sophistic and Pre-Socratic writing conventionally cited as prominent evidence for this. These treatises show all the hallmarks of being delivered in oratorical contexts, and therefore represent currently understudied evidence for the development of explanatory prose, and for the ongoing shift towards the authority of written prose over orally communicated verse or prose towards the end of the fifth century and moving into the fourth century BCE.

In Chapter 2, I considered how emphasis on Hippocratic treatises for the emergence of scientific method can obscure other layers of meaning which are integral to the persuasive aims of the authors. It was argued that as well as the surface content, or linear logic of Hippocratic expository prose treatises, other layers of 'logic', or systems or patterns of expression can be detected in Hippocratic writing and that, furthermore, there is no clear sense in the Hippocratic authors that logical systematic thinking is valued above other forms of persuasion. The chapter explored this idea through the presentation of different persuasive models in early Greek prose writing, considering the way in which logical reasoning tends to coexist with other kinds of persuasive patterning in examples from the work of Parmenides, Herodotus and Heraclitus. *On the Sacred Disease* was cited as one example of a Hippocratic treatise which both questions received wisdom about the status of the divine in relation to the 'sacred' disease using a fairly linear, logical structure, and at the same time exhibits patterning in phrasing and expression that suggest other levels of thinking and perception alongside the main thrust of the content.

The third chapter considered how Aristotle's *Rhetoric* has tended to exert a heavy influence over scholars working on early prose writing and agrees with scholars who consider this problematic; the meanings of the term *epideixis* before Aristotle's account of the epideictic genre were considered through an analysis of Hippocratic references' uses of the term. The semantic range of *epideixis* in the Hippocratic treatises focused on in this study was shown to include senses of demonstration through explanation in words and physical or visual demonstration. The term was also used in a way that hints at boundaries between areas of authority. The chapter also considered use of the term *epideixis* as a feature of the self-consciousness of the composition, and one of a variety of signposting techniques. The presence of signposting in late fifth-century oratory has been considered a feature of the orality; the dichotomy between texts designed for oral dissemination and texts for written publication was questioned, but the influence of oral composition techniques seems to be a factor in the presence of signposting features in these texts.

In Chapters 4 and 5, I went on to consider other features of orality. The fourth chapter, on the use of sound, established the point that there are clear, strong connections between *On Breaths* and earlier models of prose writing with a sophisticated use of sound patterning. Connections with Gorgias have long been established in scholarship, but here fresh analysis was undertaken: the way in which sound is being used in both treatises to echo and reinforce points being made and to serve to promote the truth value of theories was examined. Furthermore, significant connections with the Pre-Socratic philosopher Heraclitus were also established, for the same reasons. We saw how Gorgias, Heraclitus and the author of *On Breaths* all make use of structural and sonic patterns to imbue their writing with a sense of neatness and completeness, and how ideas which are central to their work are embodied in the form of the writing.

The fifth chapter explored the use of antithetical pairs in the five Hippocratic expository essays focused on in this book. Unlike previous studies of antithesis, which have sought to identify different categories of opposition, this chapter explored the resonance between oppositional pairs, and considered how the accumulation of oppositions serves to create networks of meaning underlying the surface content of the texts. It was noted that oppositions are most prominent at or near the opening of the five expository treatises, suggesting their delivery in an oral debating context and, more importantly, providing evidence for how the authors sought to use oppositional patterns creatively to establish their authority in oratorical contexts. The chains of binary oppositions are, in the opening of these treatises, a way to demarcate the parameters of a discussion, to communicate a moral position and to establish foundations on which the rest of the treatise can build.

More subtle and complex networks of oppositional pairs were found in *On Ancient Medicine* in relation to different contexts – physiology and intellectual tribalism. Here, it was seen how through layering one chain of oppositions on another, the author can convey a sense that his theory of physiology is natural and most allied with the reality of the body, and to undermine his opponents' theories and distance himself from their ideas. In place of empirical evidence, it seems that the author makes use of patterning within the body of the treatise to establish support for his claims.

We also saw how in *On the Sacred Disease*, the resonance between oppositional pairs is an aspect of the author's explanatory framework, and that though associations between oppositions does not always yield consistent points of theory, their presence has an important persuasive value that is missed if we read the treatise only for its use of linear progression of thought.

Overall, it has become clear that Hippocratic expository prose deserves to be considered, and is most fruitfully understood, as closely akin to the work of the most radical Sophistic and Pre-Socratic authors, where we find the authors searching through the medium of prose for an appropriate means to express new ideas which draw inspiration from the mythic and poetic models of authority of the past. This book has aimed to point out some of the ways in which close analysis of the persuasive strategies of these authors can yield new insights into their methods and aims; these insights serve to enhance our understanding of the extent to which a significant segment of the Hippocratic Collection contributes to the development of prose in the late fifth century BCE and shows how the medical content of their work should not lead us to think that their debates were considered rarefied or specialised in ancient times, any more than was the work of the natural philosophers, the Sophists or the early historiographers.

There is clearly much more to be uncovered from the treasure trove of evidence for early Greek prose writing that the Hippocratic Collection represents. The connections between expository prose writers and Plato's dialogues is one avenue that is beyond the scope of this book; analysis of persuasive features of Hippocratic writing which does not appear to have been designed for promulgation before an audience in a debating arena would also serve as an engaging topic for further work in this area. It is hoped that overall this book offers some convincing reasons for the importance of considering different layers of meaning and modes of communication within medical treatises and that it serves as an impetus for further research on this topic.

Appendix

Synopsis and introductory notes on the five Hippocratic 'oral' treatises focused on in this study.

1. *On Ancient Medicine*

On Ancient Medicine, as Jouanna notes, was paid little attention by ancient commentators and ironically has become one of the most well-known of the Hippocratic Collection, largely following Galen's engagement with and assessment of the treatise (Jouanna 1990: 7 f.). Mark Schiefsky's edition and translation of the treatise is the most recent, and contains an extensive introduction to the background, argument and context of the treatise (2005: 1–71), as well as a full commentary.

The treatise can be broadly split into three main sections (1-19; 20-21; 22-24). The author begins with a denunciation of the errors of medical innovators (1-2), which leads him quickly to give an account of the 'archaeology' of the discovery of medicine (2-12), followed by a return to criticism of the innovators (13-19) in which he establishes that (a) their theory that consists in attributing the cause of diseases to hot, cold, dry, humid does not correspond to reality because there is no therapy found in accordance with this (13-15) and (b) that the hot and the cold are the qualities which have the least power in the human body (16-19). In 20-1, the author abandons the polemic against the believers in hot, cold, wet and dry and explains that knowledge of the nature of man is not possible except by the study of causal relations between the regimen and the person (20), and noting that many doctors make errors because of this (21). Finally, the author gives many additional details on the causes of diseases, noting that they are due to qualities, but also to configurations of parts of the body (22-4).

The opening denunciation of medical innovators is characterised by the author contrasting the theories of those who narrow down medicine to a single primary cause (monism) with the methods and principles of medicine which the author claims have been developed over a long period. Medicine, in other words, has no need of fancy new hypotheses (2). The author claims that those who use such hypotheses and who narrow down the causes of illness to one or two primary causes fail in their approach and that they are worthy of blame, using words – 'ἁμαρτάνω', 'to fail' (1.1), μέμφομαι 'to blame' (1.1) – which are frequent in legal and tragic contexts and which highlight the agonistic setting for the treatise.

Similarly, the distinction between weak practitioners and those who excel – 'οἱ μὲν φλαῦροι, οἱ δὲ πολλὸν διαφέροντες' 'some [physicians] are bad, while others are much better' (1.2) – further entrenches this sense of binary opposition between the hero and the villain. The author is a standard-bearer and a methodologist, denigrating any deviance from the standard as deceptive and simply incorrect. In section 2, we find more language which is highly morally charged, such as 'ἐξαπατάω' 'to deceive' (2.2); similarly, deviance from this standard is evoked through the terms 'ἀποβάλλω' 'to cast off' (2.2) 'ἀποδοκιμάζω' 'to reject' (2.2), again reminiscent of legal language and criminality.

The author next explains how medicine was discovered in the first place through trial and error in searching for an improved diet (3). By searching for an improved diet, people began the process of searching for better levels of health and nourishment (3).

The author notes that the original search for a better diet cannot be classified as an art (4), but goes on to claim that certain diets were sought which were appropriate for those who were sick (5) and that it is necessary to know for whom such gruels are inappropriate (6). The author explains that the art of medicine is a development from the craft of improving diet (7) and that it can be further improved by the same techniques of trial and error (8). Doctors, we are told, must aim for correct measure in administering diets, for incorrect diets can cause harm to the healthy and the sick (9). The author notes that the most beneficial diets can be learned from the healthy (10) and that it is necessary to examine why certain diets are more appropriate than others (11). Finally, in this 'archaeology' of the art of medicine, it is stated that it is not always possible to be precise and that the art of medicine should nevertheless be marvelled at rather than cast aside.

Returning to his attack on monism, the author asks in the next section how we can tell whether, in changing the diet of a sick man to cure him, it was the hot or the cold, the wet or the dry that cured him and in preparing the bread, whether the hot, the cold, the dry or the wet has been taken from the bread (13). The author argues that, rather than powers being isolated from one another and affecting the body, foods possess a complex mixture of powers and in digesting food the body seeks to redress any imbalances, and that foods, since they are a blended mixture of powers, do not possess any single unblended and strong power but rather nourish the body with their mixture of powers (14). Indeed, the author continues, it is difficult to see how those proposing a theory of health based on the hot or the cold, for instance, can possibly treat people in accordance with this, for it is impossible to isolate one power from another.

In 16-19, it is argued that the hot and the cold, upon which theories of health are allegedly based, have least power in the body. In 16, the author describes how cold and heat can come upon and affect the body during illness, but how the body quickly responds to extremes of heat and cold and stabilises its balance of heat and cold; thus, he questions how it can be considered powerful and whether much assistance is needed against this. In 17, the author argues that the quality of being hot is always mixed with other qualities such as bitterness, acidity and saltiness; unblended qualities are said to cause illness (18), and illness is said to cease when these qualities blend again. A description of the different ways in which illness can arise, through fluxes (changes to humours) and powers is given next, with the author explaining that heat and cold in themselves are among the least powerful, easily balancing themselves out.

In the final section of the treatise (20-4), abandoning his polemic against monism, the author criticises explanations of medicine by doctors or Sophists (though this treatise itself must surely be such an explanation), claiming that it is only possible to understand disease through medicine. He explains (21) how many doctors make errors because they fail to realise that people's nature differs fundamentally and, for instance, prescribe a treatment at an inappropriate time. In 22, the author makes a distinction between powers and structures, the former meaning acuity and strength of humours and the latter meaning parts inside the human being, and notes that the structures best able to attract and draw moisture to themselves from the rest of the body are those that taper from wide and hollow to narrow, for instance the bladder, the head, and the womb in women. The author then explains how movements of air and fluids and blocks that can occur due to the internal anatomy can cause pain. Different shapes and sizes of body are said to cause different types of problem (23). The treatise concludes by summarising that it is necessary to examine what each of the humours does and its relationship with other humours and that (24) investigation from outside the body is best to discover what is the most suitable approach to each illness.

The treatise is generally thought to have been composed towards the end of the fifth century BCE (see, e.g. Craik 2015: 285; Schiefsky 2005: 63–64).

Schiefsky's translation and edition contains comments on the persuasive features of the treatise, and argues that it was originally intended for oral delivery to a lay audience (2005: 36–46) and that 'VM provides important evidence that the competitive context of ancient medicine helped to stimulate not just a tendency towards self-advertisement or exaggerated claims of competence, but also highly coherent arguments and sophisticated discussions of medical and scientific method' (2005: 45–46). I am largely in agreement with Schiefsky's insights and extensive research, but argue in this book that concerning rhetoric there are several important features of persuasive language in this treatise – such as the use of antithesis and the resonance between opposition in form and theoretical content – that have not yet been recognised by scholars and can lead us to a better understanding of the full significance of language use in the treatise.

2. *On the Nature of Human Beings*

This treatise is a critique of an understanding of human health and disease based on the notion that human beings are formed from a single element such as blood, bile or phlegm. The treatise proposes an account of the origin of human beings from a mixture of elements and argues that it is necessary for this mixture to be acknowledged and managed for health to be maintained in the human body.

The author claims that human beings are composed of blood and phlegm and yellow and black bile and that each of these elements has a nature and a power unique to it (5). The author corrects what he views as flawed observation of how physical ailments affect the body by the 'monists' and explains how each element draws to it a variety of other elements and/or qualities which make it mixed in nature (6). An account of how climatic conditions affect the balance and quality of elements in the body is given next regarding proof by experiment (7). A range of seasonal and dietetic factors, some of which are said to cause disease and others not, are then accounted for (8-9).

The author notes next that there is difference in difficulty of dealing with a disease according to whether it arose in a strong or weak part of the body (10). A description of the blood vessels in the body is given next, with the location of the vessels described as the four pairs of vessels traced anatomically (11). An account of how difference in age and lifestyle can affect the body's reaction to disease, and common changes which occur to the body through life are also outlined (12). The author reiterates the point that it is necessary to know the causes of diseases in order to cure them and gives examples of causes which are indicated through deposits and impurities in urine (14). Four types of fever are outlined ('ξύνοχος, ἀμφημερινὸς, τριταῖος, τεταρταῖος' 'unintermittent, quotidian, tertian, quartan'), and their immediate causes in terms of bodily elements (15).

There follows a second part to the treatise (16-24), which some have regarded as a separate treatise altogether (see Craik 2015: 208–211). These sections contain the following contents. Optimal diets for each of the four seasons are outlined first (16). Information on how these diets should be adapted to constitution and age is given next (17), and on how other habits such as walking and bathing should be adapted to seasons and temperaments (18). A special regimen for people who want to lose or gain weight is outlined next (19). Advice on inducing vomiting and evacuations from the lower bowels according to season and individual constitution is provided (20), followed by brief notes on good regimen for infants and women (21). Optimal regimen for athletes is outlined finally (22), with a note on symptoms of diseases of the brain and finally a moral aphorism stating that a wise man should consider health the greatest of blessings and should learn how to derive benefit from his illnesses by his own thought (23-24).

The treatise is thought to date to the last decades of the fifth century BCE (Craik 2015: 212). The most recent edition and translation is Jouanna (1990).

3. *On the Sacred Disease*

On the Sacred Disease argues that the disease commonly known as 'sacred' (thought to correspond to seizure in modern medical terminology) is no more sacred than any other disease and that it can be explained by certain physiological processes involving air and phlegm.[1]

The treatise can be split into at least four parts: (a) sections 1.1–2.1 containing an attack on those who claim that the 'sacred' disease is more 'sacred' than any other; (b) sections 2.2–13.5 containing a description in terms of physiological causes and secondary atmospheric triggering causes of the occurrence of the disease; (c) sections 14.1–17.3 containing a description of the functions of the brain and a series of claims as to its importance in the functioning of the body; and (d) section 18.1-4 containing a short conclusion.

Sections 1.1–2.1 contain an attack on the claims and procedures of the 'μάγοι' 'magi', 'καθάρται' 'purifiers', 'ἀγύρται' 'wandering priests', 'ἀλαζόνες' 'wandering quacks' and '…ὁκόσοι προσποιέονται σφόδρα θεοσεβεῖς καὶ πλέον τι εἰδέναι.' '…whoever puts on the appearance of being especially god-fearing and of having superior knowledge.' (1.4) Julie Laskaris refers to these as a group as magico-religious healers (2002 *passim.*).

Sections 2.2–13.5 of the treatise describe how humans become susceptible to the disease in the first place from improper purgation of the brain in the embryo and outline the consequences, in physiological terms, of this improper purgation. This leads into a description of the physiological cause – an abundance of 'flux' causing havoc in the body – of the attacks characteristic of the disease called 'sacred' (2.2–7.11). This explanation of the physiological causes of the disease continues with a description of how the occurrence of different quantities and qualities of flows of 'flux', often in relation to atmospheric features such as wind direction, produces different effects. The author describes the effects in small children (8.1-4), adults (9.1) and older people (9.2). In section 10, the author gives more details on the down-flows of 'flux' and the triggering causes of this in young people; in section 11 he gives details of triggering causes of down-flows of 'flux' in adults who have developed the disease in youth; in section 12, he gives details of signs indicating that the disease is about to strike and in section 13 he gives further details of atmospheric changes that can trigger the disease.

Sections 14.1–17.4 describe the pre-eminence of the brain over the functions of the body and ascribe 'mania' ('μαινόμεθα' 'we suffer from mania' (14.5)) and other mental disorders to physical changes to/in the brain. The brain is described as the interpreter of the air in section 14. Section 15 describes the functions of the heart and the diaphragm and dismisses claims that these parts of the body have any role to play in thought. Section 18 contains a statement on the author's understanding of the divine; restates the main argument of the treatise; and hints at how in principle the disease might be cured without recourse to purifications, magic and the like.

In terms of dating the treatise, Jouanna, the most recent editor of *On the Sacred Disease*, argues that the treatise can be considered as among the earliest treatises of the collection because the author does not yet know the word 'ἐπιληπτικός' ('epileptic') and does not use black bile to explain the disease, as is the case in more recent treatises (e.g. *Epidemics* 4.8, c.31; *Aphorisms* 3.20; *Regimen in Acute Diseases* section 5) (Jouanna 2003: LXXIII–LXXIV). Since black bile is probably first mentioned in *On the Nature of Human Beings* dated to 410-400, Jouanna suggests that *On the Sacred Disease* was written prior to this, and probably in the mid- to late fifth century BCE (Jouanna 2003: L, n.77; see also Craik 2015: 195).

Julie Laskaris' recent book-length study (2002) of the treatise features comprehensive analysis of the persuasive strategies of the text and examination of the notion of 'sophistic' in relation to this treatise and is an important landmark in the development of scholarship on persuasive features of the Hippocratic Collection and a major source of inspiration for this study. In her chapter of the study entitled 'A sophistic protreptic speech', Laskaris situates the treatise within the context of debates and rhetorical strategies of other treatises of the Collection that display Sophistic influence and questions the idea that the author demonstrates adherence to a clear scientific method (2002: 73–78). She claims that 'The author's primary goal is the defence of secular medicine's technical status, a project undertaken to attract clients and students' (2002: 83) and that the author adopts the Sophists' rhetorical stratagems to achieve this.

I broadly agree with Laskaris' analysis, but argue throughout this study that there is room for further and closer analysis of the use of language in Hippocratic 'oral' treatises, and that there are methods of explanation which, if not considered 'scientific method' are nevertheless significant indications of modes of thinking which tend to be obscured by focussing on features commonly related to the notion of scientific method such as an empirical attitude, and a linear progression of development of ideas. I discuss Laskaris' claims regarding the rhetoric of *On the Sacred Disease* in more detail in Chapter 5 of this study.

4. *On Breaths*

On Breaths is an exposition of the idea that air is responsible for all diseases. The treatise can be considered as split into at least two parts; namely, a well-developed prologue that offers a context for the discussion that follows, and the rest of the treatise in which the mechanics of the causation of disease by air are set forth. The first part of the prologue (1.1–1.5) describes the field of medicine, justifies its existence and to some extent portrays it as a heroic occupation that offers salvation. The second part of the prologue (beginning of 2.1 – end of 5.2) gives general principles of the functioning of the body and general ideas about what air is and of its role in the universe. Just as the first part of the prologue serves as a context and part-justification for the discussion that follows, this second part of the prologue functions as a frame in which to set the rest of the treatise, in which certain diseases are examined in turn with respect to the role of air in the causation of diseases. The second half of the prologue also lays down principles that, once accepted, give force to the argument that air is responsible for disease causation in each case that is described.

Sections 6.1–8.7 deal with the cause of the 'κοινότατος' 'most widely shared' (6.1) illness, that is fever. The author tells us that there are two different kinds of fever – epidemic fever and fever brought about by lifestyle – and he deals first with epidemic fever (6.2) and then with fever due to lifestyle (7.1f.). He discusses physiological causes of tremors (8.1-2); gaping (i.e. the opening wide of the mouth) (8.3); the relaxing of the joints (8.4); the heating up of the body (8.5); and headache (8.7).

The author notes at 9.1-2 that air must be the cause of other diseases too, citing intestinal obstruction ('εἰλεοί') and flatulent colic ('ἀνειλήματα') (9.1) and describing the cause of these disorders. He explains how air is the cause of down-flows of phlegm ('ῥεύματα') and of haemorrhage at 10.1-5. Air as the cause of lacerations is described at 11.1 and of dropsy ('ὕδρωψ') (i.e. a condition characterised by an excess of water fluid collecting in the cavities or tissues of the body). Seizures ('ἀποπληξίαι') (13.1) are dealt with at 13.1-2. The 'sacred' disease is dealt with at 14.1-7. Finally, there is a short conclusion (15.1-2) in which the author reiterates the claim that air is the primary cause of all diseases and re-emphasises its power in the universe at large.

In terms of dating the treatise, Jouanna, the most recent editor of *On Breaths*, argues that the treatise can be dated to the last quarter of the fifth century BCE on the basis that this is the era when the rhetoric of Gorgias was an admired model of prose writing, and when the monism of Anaximenes was back in fashion amongst writers on nature and medicine such as Diogenes of Apollonia (we have evidence of circulation of the idea of monism between the years 423 and 415 in the form of references in Aristophanes *Clouds* and Euripides *Trojans*) (Jouanna 1988: 48–49). Jouanna also notes that the author of the Hippocratic treatise *On the Nature of Human Beings*, which can be dated to the years 410-400 appears to refer to treatises such as *On Breaths*.[2]

5. *On the Art*

On the Art is a defence of the existence of art (τέχνη) of medicine. The author begins the treatise by exposing the polemical techniques of his opponents, whom he characterises as malicious (section 1). The tone of the opening of that of someone decrying wrongdoers and taking a moral high ground; the opening also serves as an advertisement for the art of medicine broadly speaking, while implying the existence of different approaches to and models of medicine. In section 2, the author claims that what exists cannot not exist and focuses on the distinction between reality and appearances. The author acknowledges in section 3 that the discussion on the distinction between reality and appearances (nature and convention) is part of a broader philosophical discussion and makes explicit that he is now moving on to focus on the art of medicine specifically. Section 3 self-consciously outlines and advertises that a rhetorical display will be offered in this treatise. There is a dramatic dimension to the section in the way that the author develops anticipation of what is to come as well as the characterisation of the doctor as a heroic figure, the latter recurring later in the treatise.

In section 4, the author announces what will form the focus of his discussion, that is, the distinction between luck and art. Rhetorically, the section serves to emphasise and account for the common ground between the speaker and the audience, articulating the moves towards commitment to the existence of the art by the default use of medical art: in this sense action signals belief in the existence of the art by all patients. In section 5, the author focuses on the process of understanding in medicine, noting the distinction between different abilities and levels of understanding. This contrast between expert and inexpert knowledge is a theme that recurs elsewhere in the treatise.

Again, this section suggests a wide appeal to both those who consider themselves expert and those who may not be. In the following section (6), the author notes that medicine makes use of regimen as well as drugs – once again implying that it is common to all and commonly practiced by all to some degree – and emphasises the point, with a certain amount of repetition underlining the statement, that nothing happens spontaneously. The tone of the treatise at this point is one of revealing deep and underlying truths about the nature of reality. Section 7 deals with the charge that medicine does not exist because it fails to cure fatal causes of sickness. The section is set up as in a courtroom trial, with the guilty opposed to the innocent, the guilty turning out to be the patient who 'disobeys' the orders of the doctor and follows instructions 'incorrectly'. Here, again, we have a strong moralistic and didactic stance which seeks to promote the existence of the art of medicine and deflect blame away from it by scapegoating the suffering patients.

In section 8, the author takes on the charge that physicians do not accept desperate cases. The section continues the sense of a court case taking place, with the audience as jury. The author makes clear that his opponents should distinguish between what it is possible for the art of medicine to undertake and what is not. There is a sense that the author is standing up for the art of medicine as an establishment. In section 9, the author now returns to restate the aim of his treatise and then moves on to discuss more hidden diseases, noting that medicine can tackle these too. The section also involves a comment on the kinds of people who become doctors. In section 10, the art of medicine is claimed to be a match for hidden diseases. The section then moves on to give an account of cavities in the body, outlining where these are located and describing the cells which surround the sinews running along the bones; these cells are full of juice which cause pain.

Section 11 also concerns what cannot be seen by the eyes. Patients are blamed for experiencing suffering but not knowing how to describe what they suffer. A competition between diseases and treatment is then described, with diseases said to have the advantage. The doctor is a kind of hero again in this section, if only he can 'see' what is going on within the body. In section 12, the author returns to the main argument, stating that the success of the art in dealing with obscure diseases is more surprising than its failure when it attempts to treat incurables. Such extravagant demands are not made of other arts, the author states, of which examples are given. The thread of this section is lost somewhat as the section continues to discuss the other arts.

In section 13, signs are said to appear on the surface of the body as an indication of what is taking place within. It is stated that nature can be compelled to give up secrets when they are not forthcoming. Since the relation between excretions and the information they give depends on many conditions, it is not surprising that disbelief in them is prolonged. The treatise ends (section 14) by claiming that medicine has plentiful reasoning to justify its treatment and would either refuse obstinate cases or undertake them without making a mistake. This is shown, the author states, not by attention to words but by expositions shown in acts: the crowd believes more what they see than what they hear.

The treatise is generally dated to the final decades of the fifth century BCE based on its Sophistic influence (see e.g. Mann 2012: 39–40; Craik 2015: 40).

The latest translation and edition of this treatise is by Joel Mann (2012). Mann's edition of the treatise contains detailed discussion of the text's kinship with examples of late fifth-century legal oratory; of its 'sophistic' form; and its persuasive aims and function, as well as offering a thorough overview of scholarship on this treatise relating to these topics (2012: 1–49). As with Schiefsky's discussion of the persuasive features of *On Ancient Medicine*, I am broadly in agreement with Mann's claims, but argue here that some of the richness of the persuasive features of the treatise goes unacknowledged in this edition, and that there is a dimension to the author's use of language which has not yet been well recognised in scholarship.

Notes

1 For analysis of how closely the 'sacred' disease corresponds to modern understanding of epilepsy and seizure see Temkin (1971: 15–21).
2 *On the Nature of Human Beings* opens with the lines: "Ὅστις μὲν οὖν εἴωθεν ἀκούειν λεγόντων ἀμφὶ τῆς φύσιος τῆς ἀνθρωπίνης προσωτέρω ἢ ὅσον αὐτῆς ἐς ἰητρικὴν ἀφήκει, τούτῳ μὲν οὐκ ἐπιτήδειος ὅδε ὁ λόγος ἀκούειν· οὔτε γὰρ τὸ πάμπαν ἠέρα λέγω τὸν ἄνθρωπον εἶναι, οὔτε πῦρ, οὔτε ὕδωρ, οὔτε γῆν, οὔτε ἄλλο οὐδὲν ὅ τι μὴ φανερόν ἐστιν ἐνεὸν ἐν τῷ ἀνθρώπῳ..." 'Whoever is accustomed to hear speakers discuss the nature of human beings beyond their relation to medicine will not find the present account of any interest. For I do not say that a human being is air, or fire, or water, or earth, or anything else that is not an obvious constituent of a human being...' Jouanna (1975: 165, section 1).

Bibliography

Adrados, F. R. (2005), *A History of the Greek Language*: *From Its Origins to the Present*. Leiden: Brill.

Asheri, D. *et al*. (2007), *A Commentary on Herodotus Books I–IV*. Oxford: Oxford University Press.

Audi, R. (general ed.) (1995), *The Cambridge Dictionary of Philosophy*. Cambridge: Cambridge University Press.

Auerbach, E. (1991 [1968]), *Mimesis: The Representation of Reality in Western Literature*; translated from the German by Willard R. Trask. Princeton, NJ: Princeton University Press.

Bakker, E. J., (2002), 'The Making of History: Herodotus' Historiēs Apodeixis' in Bakker, E. J., de Jong, I. J. F., and van Wees, H. (eds.), *Brill's Companion to Herodotus*. Leiden: Brill. 3–32.

Bakker, E. J., de Jong, I. J. F., and van Wees, H. (eds.) (2002), *Brill's Companion to Herodotus*. Leiden: Brill.

Barnes, J. (ed.) (1984), *The Complete Works of Aristotle: The Revised Oxford Translation*. Princeton, NJ: Princeton University Press.

Barnes, J. (1979), *The Presocratic Philosophers. Vol.1, Thales to Zeno*. London: Routledge and Kegan Paul.

Barton, J. (2005), 'Hippocratic Explanations' in Van der Eijk, Ph. J. (ed.), *Hippocrates in Context: Papers Read at the XIth International Hippocrates Colloquium; (University of Newcastle upon Tyne, 27–31 August 2002)*. Leiden: Brill. 29–47.

Beer, G. (1996), *Open Fields: Science in Cultural Encounter*. Oxford: Clarendon Press.

Bottin, L. (ed. and trans.) (1986), *Ippocrate. Arie Acque Luoghi.* Venezia: Marsilio Editori.

Buxton, R. G. A. (1982), *Persuasion in Greek Tragedy: A Study of Peitho*. Cambridge: Cambridge University Press.

Cancik, H. and Schneider, H. (eds.) (2006), *Brill's New Pauly*. Leiden; Boston, MA: Brill.

Carey, C. (2007), 'Epideictic Oratory' in Worthington, I. (ed.), *A Companion to Greek Rhetoric*. Malden, MA; Oxford: Blackwell. 236–252.

Chang, H. (2005), 'The Cities of the Hippocratic Doctors' in van der Eijk, Ph. J. (ed.), *Hippocrates in Context. Papers Read at the XIth International Hippocrates Colloquium. University of Newcastle upon Tyne, 27–31 August 2002*. Studies in Ancient Medicine 31. Leiden: Brill. 157–171.

Christ, M. (1994), 'Herodotean Kings and Historical Inquiry.' *Classical Antiquity*. 13(2): 167–202.

Clarke Kosak, J. (2004), *Heroic Measures: Hippocratic Medicine in the Making of Euripidean Tragedy*. Leiden; Boston, MA: Brill.

Cole, T. (1991), *The Origins of Rhetoric in Ancient Greece*. Baltimore, MD; London: The John Hopkins University Press.

Collingwood, R. G. (1960), *The Idea of Nature*. London: Oxford University Press.

Connors, R. J. (1986), 'Greek Rhetoric and the Transition from Orality.' *Philosophy & Rhetoric*. Penn State University Press. 19(1): 38–65.

Cooper, C. (ed.) (2007), *Politics of Orality*. Leiden; Boston, MA: Brill.

Craik, E. M. (2015), *The 'Hippocratic' Corpus: Content and Context*. London: Routledge.

Craik, E. M. (ed. and trans.) (1998), *Hippocrates: Places in Man*. Oxford: Clarendon Press.

Curd, P. and Graham, D. W. (eds.) (2008), *The Oxford Handbook of Presocratic Philosophy*. Oxford; New York: Oxford University Press.

Davies, M. (*edidit post* D. L. Page) (1991), *Poetarum Melicorum Graecorum Fragmenta*. Oxford: Oxford University Press.

Dawson, W. R. and Harvey, F. D. (1986), 'Herodotus as a Medical Writer.' *Bulletin of the Institute of Classical Studies*. Oxford: Blackwell. 33: 87–96.

Dean-Jones, L. (2003), 'Literacy and the Charlatan in Ancient Greek Medicine' in Yunis, H. (ed.), *Written Texts and the Rise of Literate Culture in Ancient Greece*, 97–121.

Demont, P. (2002), 'Équilibre et déséquilibre des 'penchants' et 'tendances' dans la médecine hippocratique' in Tacchini, I. (ed.), *Normal et le pathologique dans la Collection hippocratique: actes du Xème colloque international hippocratique, (Nice: 6–8 octobre, 1999)*. Nice: Publications de la Faculté des Lettres de Nice-Sophia Antipolis. 245–255.

Demont, P. (1993), 'Die Epideixis über die Techne im V. und IV. Jh.' in Kullmann, W. and Althoff, J. (eds.), *Vermittlung und Tradieren von Wissen in der griechischen Kultur*. Tübingen: G. Narr. 181–209.

Denniston, J. D. (1960[1952]), *Greek Prose Style*. Oxford: Clarendon Press.

Detienne, M. (1996), *The Masters of Truth in Archaic Greece*; translated from the French by J. Lloyd. New York: Zone Books; Cambridge, MA: Distributed by the MIT Press.

Dewald, C. (2002), '"I Didn't Give My Own Genealogy": Herodotus and the Authorial Persona' in Bakker, E. J., de Jong, I. J. F., and van Wees, H. (eds.), *Brill's Companion to Herodotus*. Leiden: Brill. 267–289.

Dewald, C. (1987), 'Narrative Surface and Authorial Voice in Herodotus' "Histories".' *Arethusa*. Baltimore, MD: John Hopkins University Press. 20: 147–170.

Dewald, C. and Marincola, J. (eds.) (2006), *The Cambridge Companion to Herodotus*. Cambridge: Cambridge University Press.

Diels, H. (ed. and trans.) (1964), *Die Fragmente der Vorsokratiker: griechisch und deutsch*. Zurich; Berlin: Weidmann.

Diller, H. (ed. and trans.) (1999 [1970]), *Corpus Medicorum Graecorum* I, 1, 2. *Über die Umwelt: (De aere aquis locis)*. Berlin: Akademie-Verlag.

Dodds, E. R. (1959), *Gorgias. A Revised Text with Introduction and Commentary*. Oxford: Clarendon Press.

Dover, K. J. (1997), *The Evolution of Greek Prose Style*. Oxford: Clarendon Press.

Ducatillon, J. (1983), 'Le traité Des vents et la question hippocratique' in *Formes de pensée dans la collection hippocratique: actes du IVe colloque international hippocratique (Lausanne 21–26 September 1981*. Genève: Droz. 263–276.

Ebner, P. (1962), 'Scuole di medicina a Velia e a Salerno.' *Apollo: Bolletino dei Musei Provinciali del Salernitano*. Salerno: Mondadori Electa. 2: 125–136.

van der Eijk, Ph. J. (2005a), 'The "Theology" of the Hippocratic Treatise *On the Sacred Disease*' in van der Eijk, Ph. J. (ed.), *Medicine and Philosophy in Classical Antiquity. Doctors and Philosophers on Nature, Soul, Health and Disease*. Cambridge; New York: Cambridge University Press. 45–73. [First published in *Apeiron*. Berlin: De Gruyter. 23 (1990), 87–119.]

van der Eijk, Ph. J., (ed.) (2005b), *Hippocrates in Context: Papers Read at the XIth International Hippocrates Colloquium; (University of Newcastle upon Tyne, 27–31 August 2002)*. Leiden: Brill.

van der Eijk, Ph. J. (1997), 'Towards a Rhetoric of Ancient Scientific Discourse: Some Formal Characteristics of Greek Medical and Philosophical Texts (Hippocratic Collection, Aristotle)' in Bakker, E. J. (ed.), *Grammar as Interpretation: Greek Literature in Its Linguistic Contexts*. Leiden; New York: Brill. 77–129.

van der Eijk, Ph. J. (1991), '*Airs, Waters, Places* and *On the Sacred Disease*: Two different Religiosities?' *Hermes*. Stuttgart: Franz Steiner Verlag. 119: 168–176.

van der Eijk, Ph. J., Horstmanshoff, H. F. J., and Schrijvers, P. H. (eds.) (1995), *Ancient Medicine in Its Socio-Cultural Context: Papers Read at the Congress Held at Leiden University, 13–15 April 1992*. Amsterdam; Atlanta, GA: Rodopi.

Everson, S. (ed.) (1991), *Psychology*. Cambridge; New York: Cambridge University Press.

Fallas, R. M. (2015), *Infertility, Blame and Responsibility in the Hippocratic Corpus*. The Open University. PhD thesis.

Fantuzzi, M. (1983), 'Varianza e tenacia del polar thinking nel De prisca medicina pseudippocratico' in Lasserre, F. and Mudry, P. (eds.), *Formes de pensées dans la collection hippocratique: actes du IVe Colloque International Hippocratique (Lausanne, 21–26 septembre 1981)*. Genève: Librairie Droz. 233–248.

Fowler, R. (2000–2013), *Early Greek Mythography*. 2 vols. Oxford: Oxford University Press.

Freese, J. H. (ed. and trans.) (1926), *Aristotle. Rhetoric*. London: W. Heinemann; New York: G. P. Putnam's Sons.

Gagarin, M. (2010), 'Background and Origins: Oratory and Rhetoric before the Sophists' in Worthington, I. (ed.), *A Companion to Greek Rhetoric*. Chichester: Blackwell. 27–36.

Gagarin, M. (2002), *Antiphon the Athenian: Oratory, Law, and Justice in the Age of the Sophists*. Austin: University of Texas Press.

Gagarin, M. (1998), 'The Orality of Greek Oratory' in Mackay, E. A. (ed.), *Signs of Orality: The Oral Tradition and Its Influence in the Greek and Roman World*. Leiden: Brill. 163–180.

Gagarin, M. (1986), *Early Greek Law*. Berkeley: University of California Press.

García Novo, E. (1995), 'Structure and Style in the Hippocratic Treatise, "Prorrheticon 2"' in Van der Eijk, P. J., Horstmanshoff, H. F. J., and Schrijvers, P. H. (eds), *Ancient Medicine in Its Socio-Cultural Context: Papers Read at the Congress Held at Leiden University, 13–15 April 1992* (Amsterdam; Atlanta, Ga.: Rodopi, 1995). 537–554.

Godley, A. D. (ed. and trans.) (1921–24), *Herodotus. Histories. Vol. 1*. London: W. Heinemann; New York: G.P. Putnam's Sons.

Goldhill, S. (2002), *The Invention of Prose*. Greece & Rome New Surveys in the Classics. Oxford: Oxford University Press. No. 32.

Graham, D. W. (2010), *The Texts of Early Greek Philosophy: The Complete Fragments and Selected Testimonies of the Major Presocratics*. Cambridge: Cambridge University Press.

Graham, D. W. (2008), 'Heraclitus: Flux, Order and Knowledge' in Curd, P. and Graham, D. W. (eds.), *The Oxford Handbook of Presocratic Philosophy*. Oxford: Oxford University Press. 169–188.

Greco, G. and Krinzinger, F. (eds.) (1994), *Velia: Studi e Ricerche*. Modena: Panini.

Grethlein, J. (2013), 'Democracy, Oratory, and the Rise of Historiography in Fifth-century Greece' in Arnason, J. P. *et al.* (eds.), *The Greek Polis and the Invention of Democracy: A Politico-cultural Transformation and Its Interpretations*. Chichester, West Sussex: Wiley Blackwell.

Guillén, L. F. (1992), 'Hipócrates y el discurso científico' in López Férez, J. A. (ed.), *Tratados hipocráticos: estudios acerca de su contenido, forma e influencia: actas del VIIe colloque international hippocratique, Madrid, 24–29 de septiembre de 1990*. Madrid: Universidad Nacional de Educación a Distancia. 319–333.

Habinek, T. (2005), *Ancient Rhetoric and Oratory*. Malden, MA; Oxford: Blackwell Publications.

Hall, E. (1989), *Inventing the Barbarian: Greek Self-definition through Tragedy*. Oxford: Clarendon Press.

Halliwell, S. (ed. and trans.) (1995), *Poetics* Aristotle; *On the Sublime*; Longinus; edited and translated by W. Hamilton Fyfe; revised by Donald Russell. *On style*; Demetrius; edited and translated by D. C. Innes; based on the translation by W. Rhys Roberts. Cambridge, MA; London: Harvard University Press.

Hankinson, R. J. (1998), *Cause and Explanation in Ancient Greek Thought*. Oxford: Clarendon Press.

Hankinson, R. J. (1991), 'Greek Medical Models of Mind' in Everson, S. (ed.), *Psychology*. Cambridge; New York: Cambridge University Press.

Havelock, E. A. (1986), *The Muse Learns to Write: Reflections on Orality and Literacy from Antiquity to the Present*. New Haven, CT: Yale University Press.

Havelock, E. A. (1983), 'The Linguistic Task of the Pre-Socratic' in Robb, K. (ed.), *Language and Thought in Early Greek Philosophy*. La Salle, IL: The Hegeler Institute. 7–82.

Heidel, W. A. (1941), *Hippocratic Medicine: Its Spirit and Method*. New York: Columbia University Press.

Holmes, B. (2010), *The Symptom and the Subject: The Emergence of the Physical Body in Ancient Greece*. Princeton, NJ; Oxford: Princeton University Press.

Honderich, T. (ed.) (1995), *The Oxford Companion to Philosophy*. Oxford: Oxford University Press.

Horrocks, G. C. (1997), *Greek: A History of the Language and Its Speakers*. New York: Longman.

Horstmanshoff, H. F. J. and Stol, M.; in collaboration with van Tilburg, C. R. (eds.) (2004), *Magic and Rationality in Ancient Near Eastern and Graeco-Roman Medicine*. Leiden; Boston, MA: Brill.

Hussey, E. (1982), 'Epistemology and Meaning in Heraclitus', in Schofield, M. and Nussbaum, M. (eds.), *Language and Logos: Studies in Ancient Greek Philosophy Presented to G. E. L. Owen*. Cambridge; New York: Cambridge University Press. 33–59.

Joly, R. (ed. and trans.) (1984), *Corpus Medicorum Graecorum XII, 4. Hippocrate. Du régime*. Berlin: Akademie Verlag.

Joly, R. (ed. and trans.) (1978), *Hippocrate. Tome XIII. Des lieu dans l'homme, Du système des glandes, Des fistules, Des hémorroïdes, De la vision, Des chairs, De la dentition*. Paris: Les Belles Lettre.

Jones, W. H. S. (ed. and trans.) (1947), *The Medical Writings of Anonymus Londinensis*. Cambridge: Cambridge University Press.

Jones, W. H. S. (ed. and trans.) (1998–2005 [1923–1931]), *Hippocrates I–IV*. Cambridge, MA; London: Harvard University Press.

Jouanna, J. (ed. and trans.) (2003), *Hippocrate. Tome II, 3e partie. La maladie sacrée*. Paris: Les Belles Lettres.

Jouanna, J. (ed. and trans.) (2002 [1975]), *Corpus Medicorum Graecorum* I, 1, 3. *Hippocrate. La nature de l'homme*. Berlin: Akademie-Verlag.

Jouanna, J. (1999), *Hippocrates*. Baltimore, MD; London: Johns Hopkins University Press.

Jouanna, J. (ed. and trans.) (1996), *Hippocrate. Tome II, 2e partie. Airs, eaux, lieux*. Paris: Les Belles Lettres.

Jouanna, J. (ed. and trans.) (1990), *Hippocrate. Tome II. 1re Partie. De l'ancienne médecine*. Paris: Les Belles Lettres.

Jouanna, J. (ed. and trans.) (1988), *Hippocrate. Tome V, 1re partie. Des vents; De l'art*. Paris: Les Belles Lettres.

Jouanna, J. (1984), 'Rhétorique et médecine dans la collection Hippocratique: contribution à l'histoire de la rhétorique au Ve siècle.' *Revue des Études greques*. Paris: Les Belles Lettres. 97: 26–44.

Jouanna, J. and Magdelaine, C. (eds.) (1999), *Hippocrate. L'art de la médecine*. Paris, Garnier: GF Flammarion.

Kahn, C. H. (1979), *The Art and Thought of Heraclitus: An Edition of the Fragments with Translation and Commentary*. Cambridge; New York: Cambridge University Press.

Kennedy, G. A. (1994), *A New History of Classical Rhetoric*. Princeton, NJ: Princeton University Press.

Kennedy, G. A. (trans.) (1991), *Aristotle. On Rhetoric: A Theory of Civic Discourse*. New York; Oxford: Oxford University Press.

Kerferd, G. (1981), *The Sophistic Movement*. Cambridge; New York: Cambridge University Press.

King, H. (1998), *Hippocrates' Woman: Reading the Female Body in Ancient Greece*. London: Routledge.

Kirk, G. S., Raven, J. E., and Schofield, M. (1983), *The Presocratic Philosophers*. Cambridge: Cambridge University Press.

Kneale, W. and Kneale, M. (1962), *The Development of Logic*. Oxford: Clarendon Press.

Kudlein, F. (1967), *Der Beginn des medizinischen Denkens bei den Griechen*. Zurich: Artemis.

Kühlewein, H. (ed.) (1894–1902), *Hippocrates. Opera quae feruntur omnia*. 2 vols. Lipsiae: B. G. Teubneri.

Kühn, J. -H. and Fleischer, U. (1986–89), *Index Hippocraticus*. Gottingae: Vandenhoeck & Ruprecht.

Kullmann, W., Althoff, J., and Asper, M. (eds.) (1998), *Gattungen wissenschaftlicher Literatur in der Antike*. Tübingen: G. Narr.

Kurke, L. (2011), *Aesopic Conversations: Popular Tradition, Cultural Dialogue, and the Invention of Greek Prose*. Princeton, NJ; Oxford: Princeton University Press.

Kurz, G., Müller, D., and Nicolai, W. (eds.) (1981), *Gnomosyne: menschliches Denken und Handeln in der frühgriechischen Literatur: Festschrift für Walter Marg zum 70*. München: Beck.

Lamb, W. R. M. (1914), *Clio Enthroned: A Study in Prose-Form in Thucydides*. Cambridge: Cambridge University Press.

Lanata, G. (1968), 'Linguaggio scientifico e linguaggio poetico. Note al lessico del *de Morbo Sacro*' in *Quaderni urbinati della cultura classica*. Pisa; Rome: Fabrizio Serra. 5: 22–36.

Langholf, V. (2004), 'Structure and Genesis of Some Hippocratic Treatises' in Horstmanshoff, H. F. J. and Stol, M.; in collaboration with van Tilburg, C. R. (eds.), *Magic and Rationality in Ancient Near Eastern and Graeco-Roman Medicine*. Leiden; Boston, MA: Brill. 219–276.

Lara Nova, D. (1992), 'Función literaria del prólogo en los tratados hipocráticos más antiguos' in López Férez, J. A. (ed.), *Tratados hipocráticos: estudios acerca de su contenido, forma e influencia. Actas del VIIe colloque international hippocratique, Madrid, 24–29 de septiembre de 1990*. Madrid: Universidad Nacional de Educacion a Distancia. 343–350.

Laskaris, J. (2002a), "'Acute' and 'Chronic' in '*On the Sacred Disease*'" in Thivel, A. and Zucker, A. (eds.), *Le normal et le pathologique dans la collection hippocratique: actes du Xème colloque international hippocratique*. 2 Vols. Nice: Publication de la Faculté des lettres, arts et sciences humaines de Nice-Sophia Antipolis. 539–550.

Laskaris, J. (2002b), *The Art Is Long: On the Sacred Disease and the Scientific Tradition*. Leiden; Boston, MA: Brill.

Lasserre, F. and Mudry, P (eds.) (1983), *Formes de pensées dans la collection hippocratique: actes du IVe Colloque International Hippocratique (Lausanne, 21–26 septembre 1981)*. Genève: Librairie Droz.

Lateiner, D. (1986), 'The Empirical Element in the Methods of Early Greek Medical Writers and Herodotus: A Shared Epistemological Response.' *Antichthon* 20: 1–20.

Lausberg, H. (1998), *Handbook of Literary Rhetoric: A Foundation for Literary Study*; translated from the German by M. T. Bliss, A. Jansen, and D. E. Orton; edited by D. E. Orton and R. D. Anderson. Leiden; Boston, MA: Brill.

Liddell, H. G. and Scott, R. (eds.) (1996 [1897]), *A Greek–English Lexicon*. Oxford: Clarendon Press.

Lilja, S. (1968), *On the Style of the Earliest Greek Prose*. Helsinki: Societas Humanarum Fennica.

Littré, É. (ed. and trans.) (1973–1989 [1839–1861]), *Œuvres complètes d'Hippocrate*. Amsterdam: Adolf M. Hakkert. Reprint of Paris: J.B. Baillière, 1839–1861.

Lloyd, A. B. (1975–1988), *Herodotus. Book II*. Leiden: E. J. Brill.

Lloyd, G. E. R. (1990), *Demystifying Mentalities*. Cambridge; New York: Cambridge University Press.

Lloyd, G. E. R. (1987), *The Revolutions of Wisdom: Studies in the Claims and Practice of Ancient Greek Science*. Berkeley: University of California Press.

Lloyd, G. E. R. (1979), *Magic, Reason, and Experience: Studies in the Origin and Development of Greek Science*. Cambridge: Cambridge University Press.

Lloyd, G. E. R. (1966), *Polarity and Analogy: Two Types of Argumentation in Early Greek Thought*. Cambridge: Cambridge University Press.

Lo Presti, R. (2008), *In forma di senso: l'encefalocentrismo del trattato ippocratico Sulla malattia sacra nel suo contesto epistemologico*. Roma: Carocci.

Long, A. A. (ed.) (1999), *The Cambridge Companion to Early Greek Philosophy*. Cambridge: Cambridge University Press.

Longrigg, J. (1993), *Greek Rational Medicine: Philosophy and Medicine from Alcmaeon to the Alexandrians*. London; New York: Routledge.

Lonie, I. M. (1983), 'Literacy and the Development of Hippocratic Medicine' in Lassere, F. and Mudry, Ph. (eds.), *Formes de pensée dans la collection hippocratique: actes du IVe Colloque international hippocratique: Lausanne, 21–26 septembre 1981*. Genève: Droz. 145–161.

López Férez, J. A. (1992), *Tratados hipocráticos: estudios acerca de su contenido, forma e influencia: actas del VIIe colloque international hippocratique, Madrid, 24–29 de septiembre de 1990*. Madrid: Universidad Nacional de Educación a Distancia.

Loraux, N. (2006 [1986]), *The Invention of Athens: The Funeral Oration in the Classical City*; translated from the French by A. Sheridan. New York: Zone Books; Cambridge, MA: Distributed by the MIT Press.

Lord, A. B. (1991), *Epic Singers and Oral Tradition*. New York; London: Cornell University Press.

MacDowell, D. (1990), 'The Meaning of 'ἀλαζών' in Craik, E. M. (ed.), *Owls to Athens: Essays on Classical Subjects Presented to Sir Kenneth Dover*. Oxford: Clarendon Press; New York: Oxford University Press. 287–294.

MacDowell, D. (ed. and trans.) (1982), *Gorgias: Encomium of Helen*. Bristol [Gloucestershire]: Bristol Classical Press.

Mann, J. E. (2012), *Hippocrates, On the Art of Medicine*. Leiden; Boston, MA: Brill.

Marincola, J. (1987), 'Herodotean Narrative and the Narrator's Presence.' *Arethusa*. Baltimore, MD; London: John Hopkins University Press. 20: 121–137.

Marnier, E. (1980), 'Darwin's Language and Logic.' *Studies in the History and Philosophy of Science*. Oxford: Pergamon Press. 11: 305–323.

Mayoral, J. A., and Ballesteros, A. (2001), 'Parellelism' in Sloane, T. L. (ed.), *Encyclopedia of Rhetoric*. Oxford: Oxford University Press.

Mewaldt, I., Helmreich, G., and Westenberger, I, (eds.) (1914), *Corpus Medicorum Graecorum V, 9, 1. In Hippocratis De natura hominis: In Hippocratis De victu acutorum: De diaeta Hippocratis in morbis acutis.* Lipsiae; Berolini: B.G. Teubneri.

Miller, G. L. (1990), 'Literacy and the Hippocratic Art: Reading, Writing and Epistemology in Ancient Greek Medicine.' *Journal of the History of Medicine and Allied Sciences.* Oxford: Oxford University Press. 45: 11–40.

Morison, B. (2008), 'Language' in Hankinson, R. J. (ed.), *The Cambridge Companion to Galen.* Cambridge: Cambridge University Press.

Most, G. W. (1999), 'The Poetics of Early Greek Philosophy' in Long, A. A. (ed.), *The Cambridge Companion to Early Greek Philosophy.* Cambridge: Cambridge University Press. 332–362.

Müller, D. (1981), 'Herodot – Vater des Empirismus?' in Kurz, G., Müller, D., and Nicolai, W. (eds.), *Gnomosyne: menschliches Denken und Handeln in der frühgriechischen Literatur: Festschrift für Walter Marg zum 70.* München: Beck. 299–318.

Naddaf, G. (2005), *The Greek Concept of Nature.* Albany: State University of New York Press.

Nagy, G. (2002), *Plato's Rhapsody and Homer's Music: The Poetics of the Panathenaic Festival in Classical Athens.* Washington, DC: Center for Hellenic Studies, Trustees for Harvard University; Athens, Greece: Foundation of the Hellenic World; Cambridge, MA; London: Distributed by Harvard University Press.

Nelson, A. (1909), *Die Hippokratische Schrift περὶ φύςῶν.* Inaugural Dissertation. Uppsala.

Nutton, V. (2013 [2004]), *Ancient Medicine.* London: Routledge.

O'Sullivan, N. (1996), 'Written and Spoken in the First Sophistic' in Worthington, I. (ed.), *Voice into Text. Orality and Literacy in Ancient Greece.* Leiden; New York; Köln: E. J. Brill. 115–127.

Pantelia, M. C. (ed.) (accessed Dec. 10, 2016), *Thesaurus Linguae Graecae Digital Library.* Irvine: University of California. www.tlg.uci.edu.

Parker, R. (1983), *Miasma: Pollution and Purification in Greek Religion.* Oxford: Oxford University Press.

Parry, A. (ed.) (1971), *The Making of Homeric Verse: The Collected Papers of Milman Parry.* Oxford: Clarendon Press.

Pigeaud, J. (1988), 'Le style d'Hippocrate ou l'écriture fondatrice de la médecine' in Detienne, M. (ed.), *Les savoirs de l'écriture: en Grèce ancienne.* Villeneuve-d'Ascq, France: Presses universitaires de Lille. 305–329.

Pinault, J. (ed. and trans.) (1992), *Hippocratic Lives and Legends.* Leiden; New York; Köln: Brill.

Potter, P. (ed. and trans.) (1988), *Hippocrates V.* Cambridge, MA: Harvard University Press; London: W. Heinemann.

Powell, J. (ed.) (2007), *Logos: Rational Argument in Classical Rhetoric.* London: University of London, School of Advanced Study, Institute of Classical Studies.

Purtill, R. (1995), 'Argument' in Audi, R. (ed.), *The Cambridge Dictionary of Philosophy.* Cambridge: Cambridge University Press.

Race, W. H. (ed. and trans.) (1997), *Pindar: Olympian Odes, Pythian Odes.* Cambridge, MA; London, England: Harvard University Press.

Redondo, J. (1992), 'Niveles retóricos en el Corpus Hippocraticum' in López Férez, J. A. (ed.), *Tratados hipocráticos : (estudios acerca de su contenido, forma e influencia): actas del VIIe Colloque international hippocratique (Madrid, 24–29 de septiembre de 1990)*. Madrid: Universidad Nacional de Educación a Distancia. 409–419.

Roselli, A. (ed. and trans.) (1996), *La malattia sacra*. Venezia: Marsilio.

Runia, D. T. (2008), 'The Sources for Pre-Socratic Philosophy' in Curd, P. and Graham, D. W. (eds.), *The Oxford Handbook of Pre-Socratic Philosophy*. Oxford: Oxford University Press. 27–54.

Schibli, H. S. (1990), *Pherekydes of Syros*. Oxford: Clarendon Press; New York: Oxford University Press.

Schiefsky, M. (2005), *Hippocrates: On Ancient Medicine*. Leiden; Boston, MA: Brill.

Schofield, M. and Nussbaum, M. (eds.) (1982), *Language and Logos: Studies in Ancient Greek Philosophy Presented to G. E. L. Owen*. Cambridge; New York: Cambridge University Press.

Segal, C. (1970), 'Lucretius, Epilepsy and the Hippocratic *On Breaths*.' *Classical Philology*. The University of Chicago Press. 65(3): 180–182.

Sharples, R. W. (2005), 'The Problem of Sources' in Gill, M. L. and Pellegrin, P. (eds.), *A Companion to Ancient Philosophy*. Malden, MA; Oxford: Blackwell. 430–447.

Sigerist, H. E. (1951–1961), *A History of Medicine*. 2 Vols. New York: Oxford University Press.

Singer, P. N. (trans.) (1997), *Galen: Selected Works*. Oxford: Oxford University Press.

Sluiter, I., (1995), 'The Embarrassment of Imperfection: Galen's Assessment of Hippocrates' Linguistic Merits' in Van der Eijk, P. J., Horstmanshoff, H. F. J., and Schrijvers, P. H. (eds.), *Ancient Medicine in Its Socio-Cultural Context: Papers Read at the Congress Held at Leiden University, 13–15 April 1992*. Amsterdam; Atlanta, GA: Rodopi. 519–535.

Smith, W. D. (ed. and trans.) (1990), *Pseudepigraphic Writings*. Leiden; New York; Köln: Brill.

Smith, W. D. (1983), 'Analytical and Catalogue Structure in the *Corpus Hippocraticum*' in Lassere, F. and Mudry, Ph. (eds.), *Formes de pensée dans la collection hippocratique: actes du IVe Colloque international hippocratique: Lausanne, 21–26 septembre 1981*. Genève: Droz. 277–284.

Smith, W. D. (1979), *The Hippocratic Tradition*. Ithaca, NY: Cornell University Press.

Taub, L. and Doody, A. (eds.) (2009), *Authorial Voices in Greco-Roman Technical Writing*. Trier: Wissenschaftlicher Verlag.

Temkin, O. (1971), *The Falling Sickness: A History of Epilepsy from the Greeks to the Beginnings of Modern Neurology*. Baltimore, MD; London: Johns Hopkins University Press.

Temkin, O. (ed.), and Temkin, C. L. (ed. and trans.) (1967), *Ancient Medicine; Selected Papers of Ludwig*. Baltimore, MD: Johns Hopkins Press.

Thivel, A. and Zucker, A. (eds.) (2002), *Le normal et le pathologique dans la collection hippocratique: actes du Xème colloque international hippocratique, Nice, 6–8 octobre 1999*. Nice: Publications de la Faculté des lettres, arts et sciences humaines de Nice-Sophia Antipolis.

Thomas, R. (2006), 'The Intellectual Milieu of Herodotus' in Dewald, C. and Marincola, J. (eds.), *The Cambridge Companion to Herodotus*. Cambridge: Cambridge University Press. 60–75.

Thomas, R. (2003), 'Prose Performance Texts: *Epideixis* and Written Publication in the Late Fifth and Early Fourth Centuries' in Yunis, H. (ed.), *Written Texts and the Rise of Literate Culture in Ancient Greece*. Cambridge: Cambridge University Press. 162–188.

Thomas, R. (2000), *Herodotus in Context: Ethnography, Science and the Art of Persuasion*. Cambridge: Cambridge University Press.

Thomas, R. (1992), *Literacy and Orality in Ancient Greece*. Cambridge: Cambridge University Press.

Totelin, L. (2009), *Hippocratic Recipes: Oral and Written Transmission of Pharmacological Knowledge in Fifth- and Fourth-century Greece*. Leiden; Boston, MA: Brill.

Tredennick, H. (ed. and trans.) (1933–1935), *Aristotle. The Metaphysics*. 2 Vols. London: W. Heinemann, Ltd.; New York: G.P. Putnam's Sons.

Trevett, J. C. (1996), 'Aristotle's Knowledge of Athenian Oratory' in *The Classical Quarterly*. Cambridge: Cambridge University Press. 46(2): 371–379.

Untersteiner, M. (1954), *The Sophists*; translated by K. Freeman. Oxford: Blackwell.

Van Groningen, B. A. (1958), *La composition littéraire archaïque grecque: procédés et réalisations*. Amsterdam: Noord-Hollandsche Uitg. Mij.

Verdenius, W. J. (1966–1967), 'Der Logosbegriff bei Heraklit und Parmenides.' *Phronesis* II. Assen: Van Gorcum. 12: 81–89; 99–117.

Vernant, J.-P. (1983), *Mythe et pensée chez les Grecs*. [Myth and Thought among the Greeks]. London; Boston, MA: Routledge & Kegan Paul.

Von Staden, H. (2002), 'ὡσ ἐπὶ τὸ πολύ' Hippocrates between Generalisation and Individualization' in Tacchini, I. (ed.), *Normal et le pathologique dans la Collection hippocratique: actes du Xème colloque international hippocratique, (Nice: 6–8 octobre, 1999)*. Nice: Publications de la Faculté des Lettres de Nice-Sophia Antipolis. 23–44.

Von Staden, H. (1995a), 'Anatomy as Rhetoric: Galen on Dissection and Persuasion.' *Journal of the History of Medicine and Allied Sciences*. Oxford: Oxford University Press. 50: 47–66.

Von Staden, H. (1995b), 'Science as Text, Science as History: Galen on Metaphor' in van der Eijk, Ph. J., Horstmanshoff, H. F. J., and Schrijvers, P. H. (eds.), *Ancient Medicine in Its Socio-Cultural Context: Papers Read at the Congress Held at Leiden University, 13–15 April 1992*. Amsterdam; Atlanta, GA: Rodopi. 499–518.

Wardy, R. (2009), 'The Philosophy of Rhetoric and the Rhetoric of Philosophy' in Gunderson, E. (ed.), *The Cambridge Companion to Ancient Rhetoric*. Cambridge: Cambridge University Press. 43–58.

Waterfield, R. (2000), *The First Philosophers: The Presocratics and the Sophists*. Oxford: Oxford University Press.

Watson, J. (ed.) (2001), *Speaking Volumes: Orality and Literacy in the Greek and Roman World*. Leiden; Boston, MA: Brill.

Wenskus, O. (1982), *Ringkomposition, anaphorisch-rekapitulierende Verbindung und anknüpfende Wiederholung im hippokratischen Corpus*. Frankfurt/Main: R.G. Fischer.

Worthington, I. (ed.) (2007), *A Companion to Greek Rhetoric*. Malden, MA: Oxford: Blackwell.

Worthington, I. (1996), 'Greek Oratory and the Oral/Literate Division' in Worthington, I. (ed.), *Voice into Text. Orality and Literacy in Ancient Greece.* Leiden; New York; Köln: E. J. Brill.

Yunis, H. (ed.) (2003), *Written Texts and the Rise of Literate Culture in Ancient Greece*. Cambridge: Cambridge University Press.

Index